'I was bit nervous of The GDA Diet at first. It looked like it involved a lot of maths. But as soon as I understood how to use the labels and the 20:30:30:20 rule, it was so easy. I lost nearly two stones and have kept it off. Now I use GDAs all the time when I'm shopping.'
Audrey D, Northants

'I'd buried my head in the sand for ages about my weight and what it was doing to my health. I suppose I thought that doing anything about it was just too big a task. Once I realised that just losing a couple of stones could really make a big difference it didn't seem so daunting. I'm so glad I found The GDA Diet, it's made such a difference to the way I eat.'
Matthew S, Oxfordshire

'I had a lot of weight to lose, and it had always felt like I'd got a mountain to climb to get to my target weight. Nigel's approach breaks it down into small steps, which feels so much more achievable. I'm nearly at my target now, and I just know I'm going to make it all the way for the first time in over 20 years.'
Marion M, Bromley

'I travel all over the world with my job, but the 20:30:30:20 rule means that where ever I am I'm never caught out. I just use the nutrition information panel to check the calories per serving of foods and I know I am sticking to my plan.'
Ian V, London

'The seven day plans were the perfect introduction to GDAs. I used all the 2000 calorie plans for the first three weeks; and by then I was so used to checking GDAs that I just made up my own plans and got on with it.'
Sophie D, Worthing

'Living alone means that I often don't feel like cooking complicated meals, so The GDA Diet is perfect for me. I can buy pre-prepared food, but now I am sure that what I'm eating is good for me and my diet.'
Sally W, Milton Keynes

'Although I wanted to lose weight, I couldn't stand the thought of going to a slimming club, yet I knew I needed a bit of help to learn about healthy eating. This diet has been great. It's been so simple and easy to understand and has meant I can go it alone.'
Tony B, Newquay

'These days I can't afford expensive diet food, I've got a family to feed as well myself. I loved the fact that The GDA Diet even caters for people on a budget. What a breath of fresh air.'
Sarah C, Norwich

'I knew that losing weight would be good for my physical health, but I had no idea how much it would change my emotional health too. After losing just over three stone I am more confident than I've ever been. I just seem to have a permanent smile on my face.'
Emma J, London

'When Nigel first talked to me about the diet cycle, I immediately could relate what he was saying to my own experience. I had to work really hard to break out of my own diet cycle, but now after dropping 4 dress sizes I feel fantastic and my confidence is through the roof. I know I'll never go back to my old ways.'
Caroline D, London

'The GDA Diet is the only diet I have been able to follow and maintain without getting bored. There are so many foods to choose from once you understand how to read the GDA label. It's exactly what I was looking for. Simple, straightforward and it works!'
Jackie C, London

'I lost over 3 stone with The GDA Diet and have kept the weight off for over a year. It's just become a way of life and now the whole family use GDAs to know what's inside their food.'
Libby G, Bedfordshire

'After a lifetime of yo yo dieting I've finally found an eating plan I can actually follow and I really enjoy. I'd tried every diet under the sun, but The GDA Diet is so simple and easy to follow – and it means I can eat the foods I enjoy without worrying all the time.'
Jo T, Lincolnshire

'We didn't really have too much weight to lose, but now that we're retired we wanted to start getting a bit more savvy about the food we eat. We only started using the GDAs a few weeks ago, but already we are comparing foods to see which has the least fat, sugar and salt – it makes healthy eating so much easier.'
Sue and Graham O, London

'My husband and I were able to follow The GDA Diet together. He used the 2000 calorie plan and I followed the 1700 calories plan. It was great, because it meant we could eat the same things. I just had a slightly smaller portion. Now we've lost the weight we both just follow the 2000 calorie plan and keep active and the weight stays off.'
Jen C. Kent

SHOP YOURSELF THIN
Your Supermarket Weight Loss Guide

THE
GDA
DIET

Nigel Denby RD
Dietitian and TV Nutritionist

CAPSTONE

Capstone Publishing Ltd. (A Wiley Company), The Atrium, Southern Gate, Chichester,
West Sussex PO19 8SQ, England
Telephone (+44) 1243 779777

Email (for orders and customer service enquiries): cs-books@wiley.co.uk
Visit our Home Page on www.wiley.com

Other Wiley Editorial Offices
John Wiley & Sons Inc., 111 River Street, Hoboken, NJ 07030, USA
Jossey-Bass, 989 Market Street, San Francisco, CA 94103-1741, USA
Wiley-VCH Verlag GmbH, Boschstr. 12, D-69469 Weinheim, Germany
John Wiley & Sons Australia Ltd, 42 McDougall Street, Milton, Queensland 4064, Australia
John Wiley & Sons (Asia) Pte Ltd, 2 Clementi Loop #02-01, Jin Xing Distripark, Singapore
129809
John Wiley & Sons Canada Ltd, 6045 Freemont Blvd. Mississauga, Ontario, L5R 4J3 Canada

Wiley also publishes its books in a variety of electronic formats. Some content that
appears in print may not be available in electronic books.

Library of Congress Cataloging-in-Publication Data
Denby, Nigel.
  The GDA diet : shop yourself thin : your supermarket weight loss guide : the passport to
a lifetime of permanent weight control and better health / Nigel Denby.
    p. cm.
  Includes index.
  ISBN 978-1-906465-39-1 (pbk. : alk. paper)
1. Reducing diets. 2. Food–Labeling. 3. Food–Composition. 4. Shopping. I. Title.
  RM222.2.D465 2008
  613.2'5 – dc22

                                                                    2008047082

British Library Cataloguing in Publication Data
A catalogue record for this book is available from the British Library

ISBN 978-1-906465-39-1

Typeset in DIN 9.75/13.5pt by SNP Best-set Typesetter Ltd., Hong Kong
Printed and bound in Great Britain by TJ International Ltd.

This book is printed on acid-free paper responsibly manufactured from sustainable
forestry in which at least two trees are planted for each one used for paper production.

CONTENTS

ABOUT THE AUTHOR

Nigel Denby is a registered dietitian. He trained at Glasgow Caledonian University, following an established career in the catering industry. He combines his dietetic training with a love of food – he is a trained chef and restaurateur – and has recently opened a parent/child community website www.grub4life.org.uk, which provides support, information, recipes and advice to parents and teachers of young children. He runs a practice in Harley Street where he specialises in weight management, PMS, the menopause, Irritable Bowel Syndrome (IBS) and food intolerance.

As a broadcaster for television and radio in the UK and across Europe, Nigel is a familiar face on programmes such as *The One Show* (BBC1), *Teen Mums* and *Kyle's Academy* (ITV1) and *The Truth about Food* (BBC2), and he has appeared on *BBC Breakfast* on numerous occasions. He writes for the *Sunday Telegraph Magazine*, *Zest*, *Essentials* and *Somerfield Magazine*. Nigel is also the nutritionist for www.closerdiets.com, a member of the expert panel for the 'Nutrition and Health Show' and consumer dietetic adviser for *Complete Nutrition* magazine. He is the author and co-author of seven books including *Nutrition for Dummies*, *The GL Diet for Dummies* and *Living Gluten Free for Dummies*.

In 2006 the Food Standards Agency DVD *Eatwell* featuring Nigel won a Silver Screen award at the US International Film and Video awards.

ACKNOWLEDGEMENTS

Thanks to all at Wiley Capstone, for their kindness and infectious enthusiasm for this project and for supporting my convictions.

Thanks to Tony Fitzpatrick for helping to drive the project forward, keeping everyone on their toes and dotting all the Is and crossing all the Ts.

Special thanks to Claire Loades, my colleague, right-hand woman and friend, who works so tirelessly behind the scenes and so rarely gets the credit she deserves.

Thanks to our growing band of GDA Diet supporters who have helped make this book possible. Thank you Jane, James, Gaynor, Julian, Alison, Chris and Bianca for your support, kind words, inspiration and honest, constructive feedback, which is always invaluable.

And of course, thanks to my long-suffering partner, family and friends who have been unwavering in their support ... you deserve medals!

Thank you all very much.
Nigel

PREFACE

I remember the very first time I went on a diet, I was 10 years old and joined my mum at a local slimming group. In those days it hadn't dawned on anyone that a slimming group might not be the best place to teach a 10 year old about healthy eating! Having come from a family of yo-yo dieters who loved their food and lived to eat, it seemed a perfectly natural place for me to be. I thought I was destined to be another 'fatty' in the family and so my own yo-yo dieting career began.

I have to say I wasn't very good at dieting. I suppose I thought just turning up each week would be enough; why wouldn't it be? As far as I was concerned, I wasn't fat because I ate too much and didn't take part in sport – I believed it was my fate! It felt natural for me to be shamed at my weekly meetings by having to wear a 'piggy mask' for the duration of the class because I'd put on more weight. Not only did I believe I was destined to be fat, but I also believed I was completely unable to do anything about it. I was already caught in my own 'diet cycle'.

It took another 15 years of repeating the cycle of yo-yoing between fat and thin, and being on or off a diet, before I realised fat wasn't fate, and maybe I could do something to break out of the diet cycle.

The change in my perspective happened very quickly; when I think back, it was an unbelievably easy decision to change my life path. Within three months I had given up my career in the catering industry and was enrolled on a course of five years' study to qualify as a Registered Dietitian. The more I learned about food, weight and health, the more I became puzzled that if the science made sense to someone like me (I'm not a natural academic), why was it so hard for people to put into practice?

Why were killer diseases like obesity, heart disease, cancer and diabetes soaring at a rapid rate, when making simple changes to what we eat and how we live could help to prevent them?

That was when another piece of the 'diet jigsaw' slotted into place. People are caught in their own diet cycle for reasons that are far more complex than greed, sloth, complacency or ignorance. A whole host of other influences control the choices we make, keeping us trapped in the yo-yoing cycle and usually feeling miserable.

Simply being told what's good for us isn't enough. To break free from the 'yo-yo diet cycle', we have to make changes to the way we eat that are:

▶ Permanent and sustainable
▶ Realistic and achievable
  and most importantly, they have to be
▶ Our own choices

After working as a clinical dietician within the NHS, in the world of research and in industry, I made the decision to set up my own nutrition consultancy to pursue the type of dietetics that interests me the most: preventative, permanent, realistic nutrition that empowers people to make positive changes and get what they want from life. This knowledge, combined with my personal beliefs and experience, led me to the devise the GDA Diet.

GDAs (Guideline Daily Amounts) aren't my invention; they were first introduced in the late 1990s. GDA labelling is now a familiar feature on over 20,000 of the foods we all buy, week in week out. There's nothing magical about a GDA label on its own, but the information it provides tells you all you need to know about what's inside your food, so you can make healthy choices. The GDA Diet simply explains how to use GDAs and demystifies food labels in a way that will help you to understand them – and help you to know what the information means, so you can use them to eat a healthy diet and live a healthier lifestyle.

The GDA Diet format is a powerful recipe for weight loss success and generally improved health. During the time I've been using GDAs to help my clients make more informed choices about their food, I've seen so many people who, having previously thought they'd always be stuck in their own diet cycle, have realised fantastic results in terms of weight loss, overall health improvements and the emotional gains that result from being in control of your body.

The GDA Diet incorporates everything I believe in – delicious, healthy food, flexible eating, combined with a sound scientific basis, in a simple format that is easy for everyone to use – to lose weight, keep weight off and be healthy. You really don't have to be a 'prisoner' of your weight any more – you *will* escape your 'diet cycle' with the GDA Diet.

Nigel Denby
December 2008

1 THE GDA DIET
THE DIET FOR EVERYONE

One of the questions I'm asked most often, by clients, journalists, in TV interviews or by friends, is: 'What is the ultimate diet?' Of course, the truth is there is no one diet that's perfect for everyone. The ultimate diet for each of us is the one that is safe, that works and that we can maintain for a lifetime. Each individual's diet will be slightly different, because of course we are all different.

Having said that, there are certain features that are essential for a diet to be safe, healthy and successful. The GDA Diet ticks all the 'ultimate' requirements:

► It's safe
► It works
► It suits men and women
► There are no banned foods
► It's simple and easy to understand
► There are no fancy ingredients to worry about
► The GDAs help you to adapt the way you eat to lose weight, maintain your weight loss and be healthy.
► It's an eating plan for life!

Sounds pretty good, doesn't it? Perhaps the more pertinent question to ask is: 'Why do other diets fail?'
Let me explain.

THE DIET CYCLE

We've all been there. It's Monday morning, another weekend of overindulgence is behind you, and it's D-day. You're all fired up and ready to go. You're about to start the diet! Later that week, or even that day, things may start to get a bit dodgy. You've had a stressful day at work, the kids are playing up, you're tired, hungry, haven't planned ahead for the diet, or there may be a multitude of other factors; and at that point, it's all too easy to decide the diet is just too hard or too much hassle to stick to. Your willpower slips by the wayside, leaving you feeling lousy, disappointed, guilty and like a failure.

If this sounds familiar, that's because it's exactly what I'm talking about when I describe the 'diet cycle': a cycle of preparing for a diet, starting a diet, stopping a diet, and feeling guilty about it.

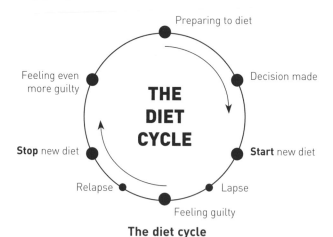

The diet cycle

When I meet a new client, we spend quite a lot of our time together talking about their previous dieting experiences. It helps us both to understand how they usually approach a diet, so we can plan a new approach that will work for them. Some of the most common reasons why clients have stopped dieting in the past include:

▶ No willpower
▶ Not enough time to bother with 'fancy' diet food

- No time to cook at all
- Can only diet when everything's going smoothly in life
- Everyone else keeps putting me off
- Stress and pressure at work
- I'm out two or three nights a week
- Diets are really confusing and complicated, I just want something simple to follow

Are these reasons for abandoning a diet, or excuses? Well, they can be a bit of both, but from my experience with my clients, and from my own dieting history, I am convinced that dieting behaviour is something we learn and can change. The more times you go through that diet cycle, the more your destructive diet behaviour becomes entrenched. The time it takes from the starting point of the diet cycle to the stopping point, and the guilty feelings of 'failure', get shorter and shorter. Eventually, for some people this means not even getting as far as starting the next diet. We come to know our personal diet cycle so well, we believe we're doomed to fail before we even start. So of course we think: 'What's the point in bothering at all?'

The most important thing to say about this pattern of behaviour is that it can all be changed: the diet cycle can be broken. The GDA Diet is a great opportunity for you to change the way you approach eating and your weight loss goals forever. Once you break the cycle you are in control, you make the decisions and you have the upper hand when it comes to changing the way you eat, look and feel.

MAKING THE GDA LEAP

Someone once taught me: 'If you do what you always did, you'll get what you always got!' So my job is to help you to take the massive and brave leap out of your diet cycle and into the brave new world of healthy living. I want to help you to break that miserable cycle forever.

Here's how it works.

The first thing you need to do is to accept and admit to yourself that you have been stuck in a diet cycle. That acceptance and understanding of what's happened in the past are *all you need* to be able to break the cycle. The new awareness gives your brain the information it needs to start afresh.

So don't waste another second beating yourself up about dieting miseries from the past. There are no 'failures', only lessons you can learn – and then you can put what you learnt into practice.

WHAT'S YOUR DIET CYCLE?

Think about the last time you started a diet that you abandoned before making the progress you'd hoped for, and work through the list of questions below to help you unravel what really happened.

I've given you a selection of answers as a starting point. Choose the answer that best fits your story, or write in your own if none of the answers is appropriate. There are no 'right' or 'wrong' answers here and you can choose as many answers as you like. This is only to help you understand your diet cycle. After you've answered the questions, read on for suggestions and tips on how to overcome and change your dieting behaviour forever.

What sort of diet did you choose?
A diet from a magazine
A diet a friend or colleague recommended
I just tried to cut down
I went to a slimming club
I always follow the same diet when I want to lose weight
Other: Write your own reason here

How did you plan for it?

I didn't
I told everyone I was on a diet and warned them not to tempt me
I filled the fridge with diet food
I just played it by ear
I cancelled my social life
Other: Write your own reason here

What did you dislike about the diet?

The food was boring
I was hungry and just thought about food all day
The diet was really confusing so I had to guess what to eat a lot of the time
It would have been fine if I was home all day, but eating out was a nightmare
I ended up cooking different meals for the rest of the family
Other: Write your own reason here

What did you like about the diet?

I got results
It was really simple and flexible
I knew exactly what to eat and when
I was dieting with a friend and we kept each other going
My friends and family were really supportive
I had clear goals I was working towards
Other: Write your own reason here

What about eating out?

I'd starve all day so I could enjoy going out for dinner
I didn't eat out
Once I started eating out it was a slippery slope
I just ordered salads
Lunchtimes were the hardest; all I could get was a sandwich
or fast food
Other: Write your own reason here

Why did things start to go wrong?

I got really stressed and gave in to comfort eating
My weight loss slowed down and I got fed up
The effort just got too much for me
I had a lapse and just couldn't get back on track
Friends and family were trying to be helpful, but they were
driving me mad going on about my diet
The weight loss was too slow; I wanted to lose weight faster
Other: Write your own reason here

**How did you feel when you realised you'd stopped
dieting?**

Relieved
Guilty
Angry and upset
It was inevitable
Hopeless
Other: Write your own reason here

OK, now you've got your answers to those questions in front of you, you can start to unravel them. Your answers are the most powerful tool you can use to help you break free from your diet cycle. They are the links in your diet cycle behaviour and they give you the keys to open the door to healthy eating and achieving a healthier body. Remember the phrase I mentioned earlier?

'If you do what you always do, you'll get what you always got!'

This is your chance to change this around to become:

'If you change what you always did, you can get what you always wanted.'

LET'S GET PHYSICAL

If you really want to be healthy and get control over your weight, a diet on its own won't work. It's really important to be active as well as to use the GDAs to help you eat a balanced diet.

But don't worry, I'm not expecting you to leap around in an aerobics class seven days a week in order to get fit. Doing simple things on a regular basis can also be highly effective, such as taking the stairs instead of the lift at work, washing the car instead of using the carwash, or cycling to the supermarket instead of taking the car. All of these can be great ways to increase your levels of physical activity without it all seeming too much like hard work.

WALK THIS WAY

Walking is easy, it's free and it's something nearly all of us can do! Regular, brisk walking can help lower your risk of heart disease and really boost your general health and wellbeing. So why not think about walking the kids to school instead of taking the car, or walking to the next bus stop on from your usual start point on the way to work?

Remember that getting fit can be fun too. Choose something really enjoyable that fits into your lifestyle: join the local netball team, go out dancing or borrow a friend's dog! Chances are, the more you enjoy it, the more you'll do it and the more fit you'll become.

GDA DIET SUCCESS SECRETS

1 Understand your own diet cycle.

2 Remember: 'If you change what you always did, you can get what you always wanted.'

3 Choose an activity that makes getting fit fun.

4 Accept your past dieting experience, learn from it and move on.

PART I
INTRODUCING
GDAs

2 CHECK, COMPARE AND CHOOSE

This chapter gives you all the background information you'll need about the GDA Diet and how it works. It also explains why GDAs make so much sense as the basis for that ever-elusive healthy balanced diet. I will explain the science behind the diet in simple terms, to help you to understand how a balanced diet leads to permanent weight control and good health.

YOU'LL FIND:

- ► A simple explanation of how the diet works
- ► The low-down on Guideline Daily Amounts (GDAs)
- ► Tips on how GDA food labels can help you lose the fat and get healthy

Let's get one thing straight: this is not a quick-fix, here today, gone tomorrow diet. The principles behind the GDA Diet are simple and based on common sense – healthy eating, combined with keeping active. It's a diet for life.

The GDA Diet is your passport to a lifetime of permanent weight control and better health.

WHAT ARE GDAs?

Quite simply, GDAs (Guideline Daily Amounts) and GDA labels take the guesswork out of knowing what we should be eating, and make planning a healthy, balanced diet as easy as pie. GDA labels allow you to control everything you eat – and that makes controlling your weight much easier.

When you ask yourself 'What do I fancy eating today?' 'What will the family want for supper?' you are also making decisions about your fat, sugar, salt and nutrient intake. Every time you go to the supermarket, you have to make decisions about health and nutrition.

Hmmm... now you know that, should you pop the pizza or the pasta in your trolley? (For the answer to that one, see page 14.) The benefit of the GDA system is that a quick glance at the GDA label on the packaging will give you all the nutritional facts you need to help you decide.

AT A GLANCE YOU CAN:

▶ **CHECK** how many calories and how much sugar, fat, saturates and salt are in your food.
▶ **COMPARE** this with something else you might fancy.
▶ **CHOOSE** the one that's right for you.

We all know that we need a certain quantity of calories a day. But if we want to keep weight at a healthy level, we can't afford to keep eating foods that give us more calories than we need. The good news is, there's GDA information about calories on almost every pack of food, to show you how many calories a portion of food contains and what percentage that is of your daily total. But calories aren't the only thing we need to keep an eye on. So there are GDAs for all the other key nutrients too, including sugars, fat, saturates and salt. (For an explanation of the function of these nutrients, please see Chapter 5.)

GDA labels give you the low-down on your favourite food and drinks

To help make life easy, over 20,000 of your favourite foods and drinks now have a GDA label on the front of the packaging, which highlights how many grams of the five key nutrients – calories, fat, saturates, sugar and salt – are in them and what percentage this is of your total daily requirement. (Strictly speaking a calorie is not a nutrient, but don't worry about that for the moment.) One quick glance at a GDA label will tell you exactly what's in the food you're about to eat. And if you look on the back of the pack, you will get other nutritional information too (see page 23).

Whatever it is you're comparing, the GDA Diet teaches you how to use the GDA food label to make the right choice. That's very good news, because let's face it, there are better things to do in life than stand in the supermarket for hours wondering what to choose for your net meal.

WHERE DID GDAs COME FROM?

Although research into GDAs has been carried out progressively over the last 20 years, they didn't appear on food labels or hit the headlines until 1998. GDA values were devised by a panel of experts from the scientific community, the food industry, as well as health and nutrition specialists (for further information see page 211). The GDA labelling system was designed to:

▶ helps consumers (that's you and me, by the way) select a better diet
▶ helps consumers make choices about the foods that suit specific needs and lifestyles

That sounds like a good recipe for healthy eating that could also help us keep in control of our weight!

The GDA label is also known as the 'What's inside?' guide. It translates the science underpinning GDAs into consumer-friendly information that can be used to make healthier food choices. By clearly showing the content of a product in per portion values, rather than per 100g, the GDA labels relate to the amount of a food people actually consume and how much of the GDAs the food contributes.

Guideline Daily Amounts were set for the nutrients we all need to eat a little less of, like fat, saturated fat, sugar and salt (these are the ones that are linked to health problems; see Chapter 5). GDA labelling is particularly useful for people who are trying to meet the GDA guidelines and puts this information in perspective. The GDAs for fat, saturates, sugar and salt are not *targets* we should aim to eat in a day, they are *maximum* amounts we should eat in a day. GDA labels make it much easier to know when we are likely to consume more than the recommended daily amounts.

There are also GDAs for important nutrients like fibre, protein and calories and these are a little more like targets to aim for. You'll always see calories on the GDA front-of-pack label, but fibre and protein don't tend to be featured on the front-of-pack labels we'll be using for the diet, although the information is still there. You can usually find fibre and protein figures when you turn a pack over and look at the general nutrition information panel on the back of the pack.

WHAT GDA PERCENTAGES MEAN

GDA stands for Guideline *Daily* Amounts. In other words, GDAs are the total, or one hundred per cent (100%), of

▶ the recommended number of calories, *and*
▶ the recommended *maximum* amounts of fat, saturates, sugar and salt that an average adult should eat *in one day*.

The figures you see on the GDA labels represent the amount of calories, fat, saturates, sugar and salt in grams that an individual food portion contributes towards your total GDA – *for one day*. The GDA label also shows the number of calories or grams per food portion and as a percentage of your total daily allowance – *for one day*. You can use either the grams or the percentages to help you keep a track of what you're eating.

Because all those numbers on your GDA label have been turned into percentages, all the hard work has been done for you. You can see at a glance how much of your Guideline Daily Amounts are in a portion of food or drink.

HOW TO USE GDAs TO CHOOSE WHAT TO EAT

You're in the supermarket, you're in a hurry, and you can't decide whether to buy a ready-made pizza or a ready-made pasta dish. Which one would the kids prefer? And which one will be better for you on your diet?

I can't answer for your kids! But if you're watching the calories, look first at the GDA label, to **check, compare and choose.**

Margarita pizza

Each 180g serving contains

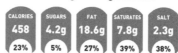

of an adults's guideline daily amount

Pasta with tomato sauce

Each 200g serving contains

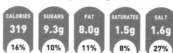

of an adults's guideline daily amount

CHECK the calories

You can see straightaway that the calorie content of the pizza (458 calories) is higher than the calorie content of the pasta (319 calories).

COMPARE the GDAs

You can also see what percentage of your total daily intake these represent. Both are within my 30% guideline for lunch and evening meal (see the diet details later in the book), but a portion of pizza, at 23%, is almost ¼ of your total GDA for the day. In contrast, a 200 g serving of pasta is only 16% of your intake.

CHOOSE what you want

If you're very hungry, you may decide that you'd rather have the pasta so you can have a larger helping! If you fancy the pizza, you know you'll have to watch the portion size more carefully.

This is a good example of how GDA labels can help you make other decisions about the food you eat. If you're trying to reduce the amount of fat or salt in your diet, you can see that the pizza contains much more fat than the pasta (27% of your GDA compared with just 11%). The pizza also contains more salt (38% of your GDA compared with just 27%). Of course, the GDA label doesn't mean you mustn't eat the pizza, but it does tell you very clearly what's inside the pizza, the pasta or any other food.

The GDA label allows you to check, compare and choose the best food for you and your health. (Remember to avoid adding extra salt, fat or sugar to food once you've served it up, though!)

You can use GDAs to keep track of calories or you can use them to keep a track of all of the key nutrients in your food.

1 The GDA Diet is a diet for life.

2 GDA labels take the guesswork out of planning a healthy, balanced diet.

3 Use GDA labels to CHECK the calories, COMPARE the GDAs and CHOOSE what you want.

4 GDA labels will help you spot when you've had too much of a good thing.

3 HOW TO READ YOUR GDA LABELS

The average daily adult requirement for calories is considered to be approximately 2000. So, when you look at the calories on a GDA label, they are calculated on the basis of an average of 2000 calories per day.

2000 calories = 100% of your GDA *per day*.

Now you know that, the rest is easy.

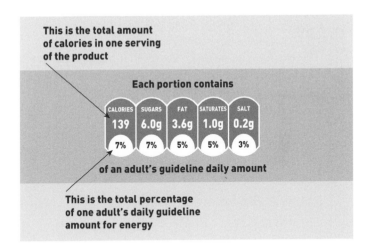

This is the total amount of calories in one serving of the product

Each portion contains

CALORIES	SUGARS	FAT	SATURATES	SALT
139	6.0g	3.6g	1.0g	0.2g
7%	7%	5%	5%	3%

of an adult's guideline daily amount

This is the total percentage of one adult's daily guideline amount for energy

%   This is the percentage of your GDA for the calories you're about to eat.

Calories   This figure tells you how many calories there are in 1 portion of your food.

%	This is the percentage of your GDA for the sugars you're about to eat.
Sugar	This figure tells you how many grams of sugar are in 1 portion of your food.
%	This is the percentage of your GDA for the fat you're about to eat.
Fat	This figure tells you how many grams of fat are in 1 portion of your food.
%	This is the percentage of your GDA for the saturates you're about to eat.
Saturates	This figure tells you how many grams of saturated fats are in 1 portion of your food.
%	This is the percentage of your GDA for the salt you're about to eat.
Salt	This figure tells you how many grams of salt are in 1 portion of your food.

The example on page 17 shows that a single portion of the product contains 139 calories. It also shows that 139 calories are 7% of your total GDA.

If you're buying a pre-packed ready meal, the important thing to remember is:

CHECK HOW MANY PORTIONS THE PACK IS MEANT TO FEED.

Whether it says Serves 1, 2, 3, 4 or more, REMEMBER that the label shows the measurement for just ONE of those portions. It's easy to eat double or triple portions if you don't take care when it's time to serve up.

Eating well is definitely a balancing act! Getting to know which foods you should eat plentifully and which foods you should limit to 'every now and then' will require a bit of thought and planning. GDA labels are especially useful because they don't just show you what's in the product you're about to eat. They also tell you how a portion of that food or drink will fit your daily diet plan. Use GDAs to help you to get the balance right.

The GDA eating plans and GDA food lists included in Chapters 8 and 9 have been carefully planned to make sure you are getting the right balance of everything you need to be healthy while you lose weight.

Getting to know your GDAs and using them as a guide can help you to control your overall diet more effectively. For example, if you choose to eat something at lunchtime that's a bit high in fat, you can balance this out at dinner by choosing a low-fat meal. Similarly, if you're going to go out for dinner and you know you won't be able to resist a sweet pudding, then throughout the day you can choose foods that don't contain a lot of sugar and there's no harm done.

Keeping an eye on GDA labels means you'll never be fooled into thinking a food is good for you when it's really full of hidden sugar or fat; and conversely, you'll never miss out on eating something you think might not be so good for your waistline, when the GDA label shows you that the ingredients are good for you instead.

In short, GDA labels open your eyes to the foods on the supermarket shelves. The GDA Diet is the only tool you'll ever need to make balanced food choices and stay on the right side of healthy, great tasting, convenient food.

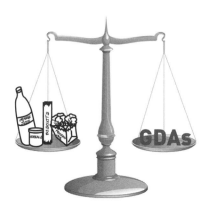

All the diets I'd ever tried before were about banning foods. At last there's a diet which teaches me how to balance my food – it just makes so much sense!
Pauline W, Surrey

INTRODUCING THE 20 : 30 : 30 : 20 RULE

To help you keep track of what you're having throughout the day, it's useful to split your GDAs into meals and snacks. I recommend the following breakdown:

Breakfast:	20% of your GDA
Lunch:	30% of your GDA
Evening meal:	30% of your GDA
Snacks:	20% of your GDA

You don't need to be too exact about this: think of it as a rough guide. If you go over target on a nutrient such as fat at one meal, then just choose a lower-fat option later. I usually recommend that snacks are divided into two: one in the morning (10%) and one mid-afternoon (10%). This has the benefit of keeping your blood sugar on an even keel so you reduce hunger pangs and food cravings. Eating three meals and two snacks a day, at regular intervals, is commonly recommended by dietitians and other health professionals when helping people to control their weight.

The 20:30:30:20 rule is explained in more detail in Chapter 6 on planning. And all the thinking has been done for you in the 7-day diet plans (Chapter 8).

I don't want you to worry about remembering grams and percentages. That's just too much like hard work! As a general guide, *avoid foods that are high in saturates and sugar* and keep in mind the number of calories you're aiming for at each meal and snack.

ALL KINDS OF FOOD LABELS

Many of you may be wondering why GDA labels aren't on *all* the foods you buy. In the UK we currently have two types of labelling on the front of food packs: GDAs and Multiple Traffic Lights (MTLs). The traffic lights show you red, amber or green symbols for fat, saturated fat, sugar and salt. They don't always include a symbol for calories. Traffic lights act as a general 'warning' system. They show only the coloured symbol, not the actual amount of fat or sugar that's inside the food, so I don't think they make it as easy to keep a track of what you eat throughout the day.

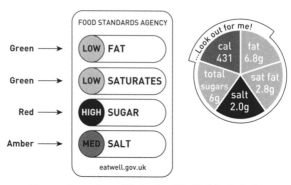

Examples of multiple traffic lights labels

Some people like the traffic light labels because they show 'the good, the bad and the ugly' food types by colour. However, they don't include the percentages. This leads us to think about each food in isolation, rather than in the context of all the other foods we eat throughout the day, and of course a healthy balanced diet needs to consider all of the foods we eat.

A food with a traffic light label can still be part of your GDA Diet. If you flip over to the back of the pack you will nearly always find the GDA information as part of the nutrition information panel. So all you need to do is check the amounts against the 20:30:30:20 values according to when you're planning to eat the food as breakfast, lunch, dinner or as a snack.

Margarita pizza

Nutrition

Typical values	100g contains	Half of a pizza (172.5g) contains	%GDA*	GDA* for a typical adult
Energy	1020kJ 245kcal	1760kJ 420kcal	21%	2000kcal
Protein	11.5g	19.8g		
Carbohydrate	29.9g	51.6g		
of which sugars	3.2g	5.5g	6%	90g
Fat	8.5g	14.7g	21%	70g
of which saturates	4.4g	7.6g	38%	20g
mono-unsaturates	2.5g	4.3g		
polyunsaturates	1.0g	1.7g		
Fibre	1.2g	2.1g		
Sodium	0.3g	0.5g		
Salt equivalent	0.7g	1.2g	20%	6g

*Guideline daily amounts

Example of a back-of-pack nutrition label showing Guideline Daily Amounts (GDAs)

Some manufacturers and retailers use a combination of traffic lights and GDAs in what's called a 'hybrid' label. These labels combine a traffic light colour – green, amber or red – as well as the GDA values. If you're contemplating one of these labels to help you decide if you want to include the food in your GDA Diet, then just look at the GDA value in the normal way.

SERVES 2 - HALF PACK PROVIDES				
CALS 390	SUGAR 2.7g	FAT 26.4g	SAT FAT 12.5g	SALT 1.68g
20%	3%	38%	62%	28%

OF YOUR GUIDELINE DAILY AMOUNT

Example of a hybrid food label showing calories and grams, but not GDA percentages

While it may seem a bit crazy that retailers use several different labelling systems, don't be put off. By following the GDA Diet approach you'll be able to get the information you need wherever you shop and whatever you buy. Just CHECK, COMPARE and CHOOSE by looking at the GDA percentages.

CAN YOU TRUST WHAT THE LABEL SAYS?

Some foods make claims to be a good source of a particular nutrient (e.g. 'high fibre') or to contain more or less of the nutrient than a standard item (e.g. 'low fat' or 'low in sugar'). These claims are useful signposts for the busy consumer, but what do 'low' and 'high' actually mean?

Manufacturers are obliged to stick to certain guidelines to avoid making claims that may mislead us. The definitions are still being standardised, but the general consensus is summarised in the table below.

Guidelines for Nutritional Claims per 100 g or 100 ml

Nutritional claim	Definition
Low calorie	40 kcal or less (10 kcal for drinks)
Low sugar	5 g or less
Low fat	3 g or less
Low sodium	40 mg or less
Reduced sugar Reduced fat Reduced salt	Contains at least 25 per cent less than standard product
Sugar free	0.2 g or less
Fat free	0.15 g or less
High fibre	6 g per 100 g or at least 3 g of fibre per 100 g

Some foods that claim they are low sugar, for example diet drinks, may contain substitute ingredients like artificial sweeteners in order to make the claim but still taste sweet. Other foods like low-sodium breakfast cereal will simply use less salt in the production process. The ingredients list will often give you an idea if a substitute ingredient has been used.

THE GDA DIET IS UNIQUE

The GDA Diet uses GDA labels to balance your food intake, and includes all the fruit, vegetables, oily fish, beans and pulses you'll ever need. We mix in a little physical activity too. (Please note I didn't say exercise.) The result is a lifestyle and eating plan that allows you to buy and eat the food you know and like, wear the clothes you want in the sizes you like, – and stay healthy too.

If you've ever wanted a simple, one-stop reference to common-sense healthy eating that also allows you stay in charge of your waistline, then look no further! The GDA Diet is the answer you've been looking for.

Once you know what's inside your food, you can CHECK, COMPARE and CHOOSE what to buy and what to eat. Once you can do that, you're always in the driving seat and always in control of what you eat.

Have a look at page 225 – and the GDA Diet website, www.gdadiet.com – for the latest list of all the manufacturers and retailers who use GDA front-of-pack labels.

1 Make sure you understand how to use the GDA labels.

2 Be aware of other kinds of food labels.

3 Know the 20:30:30:20 rule.

4 Choose the GDA diet plan that's right for you and factor in a little extra physical activity.

PART II
YOUR GDA
LIFESTYLE

4 GDAs AND YOUR HEALTH

This chapter helps you to decide which GDA diet plan will be right for you, and explains the role of the nutrients that you see on the GDA labels. I want to help you to understand how keeping control of the total amount of fat, saturated fat, sugar and salt you eat can reduce your risk of poor health later in life.

What's useful about GDA labels is that they not only help us watch calories (which is of course the central issue surrounding weight control), but they also help us to keep tabs on the things we *all* need to eat a little less of, if we're to stay healthy.

HOW GDAs HELP IN WEIGHT CONTROL

Eating too much fat, especially saturated fat, sugar and salt is bad news for the body. Fatty and sugary foods are high in calories and can lead to weight gain when eaten in excess, and too much salt in the diet is linked to an increased risk of high blood pressure. But of course, the problem is that fat, sugar and salt make food taste great. We don't need to cut all of the fat, sugar and salt out of our diets – in fact if we did that wouldn't be healthy either. It's all about balance.

When we get the nutritional balance wrong and eat too many fatty, sugary foods and salty snacks, it speeds up weight gain because these foods are usually high in calories. (These sorts of foods don't tend to contain many vitamins and minerals either, so if we eat too many of them we can miss out on a whole host of nutrients that we need to be healthy.)

Suddenly those jeans don't look quite as good as they did; the shirt starts to gape open at the buttons, and the love handles wobble when we walk. We all know the feeling! This is where GDAs can be your best friend. They will help you to keep track of how much you're eating and also remind you of how much is too much. The pack labels tell you instantly the amount of fat that's in that portion of pie, and what percentage that amount of fat contributes to your GDA for the day. You can't duck the facts once you know where to look!

WHICH GDA PLAN IS RIGHT FOR YOU?

GDAs have been developed for men, women and children from 5 upwards. However, if you have a child who needs to lose weight, instead of following the guidelines in this book please go to your GP for advice.
This book is about GDAs and weight control for adults.

I use two sets of GDAs that will help you lose weight and keep it off. But before you decide which plan is right for you, it's important that you take stock and decide what your starting point is. If you're not sure how much weight you need to lose, check out 'How do you shape up?' on page 33.

Do you need to lose more than 13 kg (2 stone) in weight?

For most men and those women who have 13 kg or more to lose, the GDA values used as a basis for the labels on over 20,000 food packs are enough to create a perfect diet for you.

Following the 20:30:30:20 guide (see page 20) will ensure you consume a maximum of 2000 calories a day, and the right amount of fat, saturates, sugar and salt to be healthy. With a fairly modest amount of activity each day (30–40 minutes) you should be able to lose a safe, steady and maintainable ½-1 kg (1–2 lb) per week.

Weight loss GDAs for those who need to lose less than 13 kg (2 stone)

I know it might not seem like it to you at the moment, but if you're less than 13 kg overweight, you have only a modest amount of weight to lose. But that's no reason for complacency. Remember – rather like shares and investments – your weight can go up as well as down!

You need to be a little more careful about the level of calories you eat each day. Eating food to a total of around 1700 calories a day, and combining this approach with a little activity, will be just fine to help you lose a safe, steady and maintainable amount of weight: ½–1 kg (1–2 lb) per week. You still need to eat plenty of the nutritional goodies, so we'll focus on reducing your calories from fat and sugar to make sure you don't miss out.

You may be wondering why I'm advising people who need to lose more weight to eat a higher number of calories than those who have a relatively modest amount of weight to lose. It's because heavier people need more calories than lighter people for their bodies to function properly. This a healthy weight loss plan, not a crash diet, so it's important that you make sure your diet allows you to lose weight but also gives you the energy and nutrients you need to be healthy.

If you're following the 1700-calorie plan, then you'll need to CHECK, COMPARE AND CHOOSE from the actual figures for calories and grams of fat and sugar rather than percentages. This is because the percentages on the GDA labels relate to a diet based on 2000 calories per day; they show the amount of fat and sugar as a percentage of 2000 calories. Your eating plan provides you with 1700 calories, so the actual number of calories and the grams of fat, saturates and sugar are the important figures that will keep you on track.

You still divide your calories up throughout the day using the 20:30:30:20 rule (see page 20), but your breakfast will provide 20% of 1700 calories (340 calories). That's only 60 calories less than on the 2000 calorie plan.

Should I count actual values or percentages or both?

If you're following the 1700-calorie plan, you'll need to focus on the actual figures for calories, fat, saturates, sugar and salt.

People using the 2000-calorie plan can tot up the percentages – or the actual gram weights – for foods they eat during the day. Remember: the main sources of calories in your diet are fat and sugar. But on either plan, don't forget to factor in the calories that are in your drinks and snacks as well as those in your meals. (See tips on saving drinks calories on page 42).

MORE CHOICE WITH THE GDA DIET

We all lead different lives, we all like to eat different things and what we choose to eat can be affected by outside influences like time, money or personal beliefs. So I have taken the GDA Diet plans a stage further. As well as plans to suit men and women with different amounts of weight to lose, I have made plans for you to choose from according to the sorts of foods you like to eat:

The plans for busy people are for people who rarely cook for themselves: they are based entirely on convenient, prepared foods you can find in any supermarket or on any high street.

The plans for vegetarians are exactly what they say: meat-free zones

The plans for people on a budget are just as nutritious as the other plans, but keep an eye on the pennies as well as the calories and other key nutrients.

Once you decide whether you need to follow the 2000-calorie or 1700-calorie plan, you can swap between the plans for busy people, vegetarian plans or plans for people on a budget, or if you prefer you can choose one plan and one calorie allowance and follow it to the letter. It's up to you. Just don't make the mistake of swapping between the 2000-calorie and 1700-calorie plans because they have been designed for different weight loss requirements.

No foods are banned on the GDA Diet. The choices are all yours. GDAs help you to control the *amount* of food you buy that contains high levels of 'not-so-good' nutrients (i.e. saturated fats, sugar and salt) and to balance these with the right quantity of foods containing the nutrients we really need (i.e. vitamins, minerals and fibre, as well as protein). The body needs these nutrients, and a certain level of calorie-driven energy, to function properly and repair itself.

If you fancy something a little indulgent, something that's got more calories, sugar or salt in it, than you should be having it as part of the 20:30:30:20 guide. It's not a problem, just make sure that your *total* percentages for the day stay roughly within (or below) 100 per cent. So keep an eye on the GDA percentages on your labels. That way you'll be able to gauge for yourself what you're eating throughout the day. If you decide to treat yourself, simply try not to overdo it with the rest of your meals for the day.

Of course, this doesn't mean it's okay to starve yourself all day just so that you can have a huge piece of gâteau for dinner! You need to eat at regular intervals to be healthy and to give yourself the energy you require to go about your daily business. A treat is something you have occasionally, when you're out for dinner or celebrating a birthday – not every day.

HOW DO YOU SHAPE UP?

Are you a healthy weight for your height? About 1 in 5 adults in the UK today are heavy enough to be putting their health at risk. There are several ways of checking whether your current weight or body shape is likely to affect your health. These include working out your Body Mass Index (BMI) and checking your waist size. Please note the measurements given here are for adults over 18 years.

Calculate your Body Mass Index (BMI)

Measuring your Body Mass Index (BMI) is a useful way of finding out whether your weight is putting your health at risk. Your BMI, a measure that is used by health professionals around the world, is based on your height and weight and can be worked out by dividing your weight (in kilograms) by your height (in metres) squared.

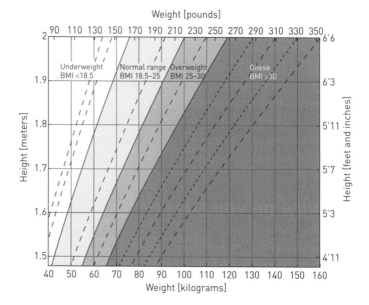

For any height there is a range of healthy weights. BMI is classified in the following way:

▶ **Less than 18.5 kg/m²** You are underweight. You may need to gain weight. GDAs may be helpful as a guide to check whether you're eating enough, but you shouldn't be trying to lose weight.

▶ **19 to 24.9 kg/m²** You are a healthy weight and should aim to stay that way. GDAs can be used to help you maintain your healthy weight or lose just a small amount of weight.

▶ **25 to 29 kg/m²** This level of BMI is defined as overweight. It's a good idea to lose some weight for your health's sake, or at least aim to prevent further weight gain. A good target for weight loss for you will be between 6.5 kg–13 kg (1–2 stone) over 3–4 months.

▶ **Over 30 kg/m²** This level is defined as fat and your health is at risk. Losing weight will improve your health. A good initial target for weight loss would be 13 kg (2 stone), although you may need to lose a little more than this to achieve a healthy BMI.

▶ **Over 35 kg/m²** You should visit your GP for a health check, as you may need specialist help to manage your weight and health. This is especially important before taking up any new exercise.

Note: BMI is not always a good reflection of body fatness. A very muscular person might have a high BMI when in fact their body fat is at a healthy level, as muscle weighs more than fat.

Have a look at the BMI chart page 34 and plot where you are right now:

▶ If your current BMI is between 22 and 25, then you'll need to follow the 1700-calorie GDA plan because you should only be aiming to lose a moderate amount of weight. You can expect a weekly weight loss of about 1 kg (1–2 lb). Weight loss tends to be slower the less you need to lose.

▶ If your BMI is between 20 and 22, be careful that you don't lose too much weight. A low BMI below 18.5 can be just as unhealthy as being overweight.

▶ If your BMI is between 25 and 30, or you're a man who needs to lose some weight, you'll be following the 2000-calorie plan and could expect to lose a little more each week to start with.

▶ If your BMI is above 30, you'll be following the 2000-calorie plan and it wouldn't be unusual to lose up to 2 kg (5 lb) in 7 days, especially if you're able to be more active than usual, but check this first with your doctor. This kind of early, rapid weight loss will slow down as your body gets used to your new routine.

Waist measurements and what they mean

It would also be a good idea to take some measurements like waist, hips and bust or chest. Use a flexible tape measure and make sure you measure the same spot each time. Keep the tape measure straight for the most accurate results.

▶ Waist – measure around the naval or belly button
▶ Hips – measure at the widest point of your bottom
▶ Bust or chest – measure around the widest point

Waist measurement is a good indicator of your fat distribution, which is linked to health risk. Carrying too much weight around your middle is a sign that you're at increased risk of developing heart disease, high blood pressure and diabetes.

People who carry excess weight around their middle are often referred to as 'apple shaped', whereas those who carry the weight on their hips are 'pear shaped'. Women are usually pear shaped, while men are more likely to be apple shaped. Measuring your waist is an easy way of finding out whether you're an 'apple' or a 'pear'.

Use the table below to see if you are at risk of ill health. Remember, these measurements refer to adults, not children.

Waist measurement

	At increased risk	*At high risk*
European men	94 cm (37 in) Aim to lose between 1 and 2 stones (6.5 kg to 13 kg)	102 cm (40 in) Aim to lose at least 2 stones (13 kg)
Asian men	90 cm (36 in) Aim to lose between 1 and 2 stones (6.5 kg to 13 kg)	96 cm (38 in) Aim to lose at least 2 stones (13 kg)
All women	80 cm (32 in) Aim to lose between 1 and 2 stones (6.5 kg to13 kg)	88 cm (35 in) Aim to lose at least 2 stones (13 kg)

If you are at increased risk, now would be a good time to make healthy lifestyle changes that would reduce or prevent any further increase. If you are at high risk, then losing weight and reducing your waist size would improve your health.

If you are working to increase your day-to-day activity levels, then measurements will be especially important to you, because you may well change shape and lose inches faster than you lose weight. This is because as you increase your activity level, you replace some fat with muscle, and muscle is heavier than fat. This increase in muscle tissue is exactly what you want. More muscle tissue results in a faster metabolic rate and that means you burn more calories even when you're asleep. And, you guessed it, burning more calories means that you lose weight more easily!

A general guide for a healthy weekly weight loss is between ¼ kg and 1 kg (½ lb to 2 lb a week) or anything up to 1 kg per week.

However you use GDAs, the main thing is to find a system that works for you. That way, you're much more likely to stick with your diet plan and keep things under control.

1 Eating too much fat, sugar and salt is bad for your health.

2 Calculate your BMI and check your waist size.

3 If you need to lose more than 13 kg (2 stone), follow the 2000-calorie plan.

4 If you need to lose less than 13 kg (2 stone), follow the 1700-calorie plan.

5 If you're busy, a vegetarian or on a budget, there's a plan that's right for you.

6 A healthy weekly weight loss is up to 1 kg per week.

5 CALORIES, SUGARS, FATS, SATS, SALT – AND YOU!

GDA labels feature five key nutrients and you've seen and heard about all of them before. But do you know why it's good to keep below the recommended GDA for salt? Or why fat is needed at all? Or why we need to keep tabs on the amount of added sugar we eat? This chapter gives you the facts behind the figures.

CALORIES

Calories are not your enemy. Calories are a unit of energy. They are used to measure how much energy your food provides and your body needs to allow your heart to beat, your lungs to breathe and your body to heal and repair itself when it's damaged. Without burning calories you couldn't get up and move about – in fact you couldn't think or function at all. But the energy you take in from food and drink needs to come from all the food groups, so you get the right mix of vitamins, minerals and other nutrients you need. There are many aspects that make up a healthy diet, including fibre from wholegrains and pulses, calcium to keep bones healthy, protein to help our bodies heal and repair, and fluid to transport all these nutrients to the places they need to go. Planning a balanced diet means that you can keep track of where your calories come from.

That's the secret of the elusive healthy balanced diet that people like me are always talking about.

"Both my parents have Type II diabetes and with the extra three stone of weight I was carrying my doctor said I was a dead cert to follow in their footsteps. Now I'm losing the weight and getting fitter he says I have nearly halved my chances of getting it. I couldn't change my genes, but I could change my lifestyle; and GDAs really helped me get a handle on what I was eating."
Sean G, Hertfordshire

SUGARS

Sugar gives the body energy and, of course, helps make sweet foods taste good. The sugars in our diet come from lots of different sources: some of them are obvious, like the refined white sugar you sprinkle on cornflakes or stir into a cup of tea; others are less obvious and can be lurking where you might not expect to find them. For example, there are naturally occurring sugars in things like fruit, fruit juice and milk, or more complex carbohydrates which the body breaks down is sugar in foods that we don't necessarily think of as being sweet, like baked beans, tomato ketchup or bread and pasta.

While most of us like the taste of having *some* sugar in our diet, it's important to stay within your Guideline Daily Amount. Too much sugar is bad news for your teeth and your waistline. The sugar that occurs naturally in foods like fruit and milk is less of a problem, because it arrives with a whole host of other nutritional goodies such as antioxidant vitamins (A, C, E and beta carotene) and calcium. The sugar to be wary of is the white stuff and the hidden sugars. Nutritionists and dietitians tend to class added sugar as 'empty calories' – that's calories which don't provide any other real nutritional benefits. Empty calories = added body fat.

The GDA for sugars for an adult consuming 2000 calories a day is 90 g.

The GDA for sugars for an adult consuming 1700 calories a day is 76.5 g.

Most adults in the UK eat too much sugar, so we should all be trying to eat fewer sugary foods, such as sweets, cakes and biscuits, and to drink fewer soft drinks.

Sugar is added to many types of food, such as:

▶ fizzy drinks and juice drinks

▶ sweets and biscuits

▶ jam

▶ cakes, pastries and puddings

▶ ice cream

What about fruit juice?

The sugars found naturally in whole fruit are less likely to cause tooth decay than are refined sugars because they are contained within the structure of the fruit. But when fruit is juiced or blended, the sugars are released. Once released, these sugars can damage teeth, much like other sugars, especially if fruit juice is drunk frequently.

Fruit juice is a healthy GDA choice and counts towards the five portions of fruit and vegetables we should be having every day, but it is best to drink fruit juice at mealtimes and stick to one small glass per day.

Tips for cutting down on your sugar intake

If you have a sweet tooth and are trying to reduce your sugar intake, these tips might help you cut down:

▶ Have fewer sugary drinks and snacks.

▶ Instead of sugary fizzy drinks and juice drinks, choose water or unsweetened fruit juice.

▶ If you like fizzy drinks, then try diluting fruit juice with sparkling water.

▶ Instead of cakes or biscuits, try having a currant bun, scone or some malt loaf with low-fat spread.

▶ If you take sugar in hot drinks, or add sugar to your breakfast cereal, gradually reduce the amount until you can cut it out altogether. Eventually your taste buds won't miss it.

▶ Rather than spreading jam, marmalade, syrup, treacle or honey on your toast, try a low-fat spread, sliced banana or low-fat cream cheese instead.

▶ Use GDA labels to help you CHECK, COMPARE and CHOOSE the foods with less added sugar.

▶ Try halving the sugar you use in your own recipes. It works for most things.

▶ Choose tins of fruit in juice rather than syrup.

▶ Choose wholegrain breakfast cereals or porridge rather than those coated with sugar or honey, or try a mix of half and half.

What if there are no GDAs on the pack?

You can get a feel for whether a product is high in added sugars by looking at the ingredients list.

Added sugars must always be included in the ingredients list, which starts with the biggest ingredient. Watch out for other words that are used to describe added sugars, such as sucrose, glucose, fructose, maltose, hydrolysed starch and invert sugar, corn syrup and honey. If you see one of these near the top of the list, you know that the product is likely to be high in added sugars.

TOTAL FAT

A healthy diet should always include a certain amount of fat because, among other things, fat provides energy and helps you absorb vital vitamins. There are also special, essential fats, which we can only get from foods. Fat makes our food feel nice in our mouths, which is why crispy chips or chocolate are such a temptation. But of course, too much of a good thing becomes a problem.

Fat contains more calories per gram (9 calories per gram) than any other nutrient, so a diet that is high in fat will also be high in calories, which will make it more difficult to control your weight.

Try to eat no more than your Guideline Daily Amount and choose unsaturated fats as often as possible. Unsaturated fats are the ones you find in oily fish, nuts and seeds, avocado and sunflower, rapeseed or olive oil.

The GDA for fat for an adult consuming 2000 calories per day is 70 g.

The GDA for an adult consuming 1700 calories per day is 60 g.

Individual GDAs for both fat and saturates are shown on the GDA labels. The GDA figure for fat is the *total* amount of fat a food contains, *including* saturates and unsaturated fat (see below). Saturated fat is the type of fat most commonly linked to health problems like heart disease, which is why it is highlighted separately on the GDA labels as well as being included in the overall total GDA for fat.

Different sorts of fat

We should be cutting down on food that is high in saturated fat or trans fats, or replacing these foods with those that contain unsaturated fat (polyunsaturated and monounsaturated fat) instead. We should also be having more omega-3 fatty acids, which are found in oily fish.

SATURATED FAT

Food that contains lots of saturates, such as pastries, butter, cheese and cream, may taste great, but when we eat too much saturated fat it can raise blood cholesterol, which increases the risk of heart disease.

Avoid having more than the Guideline Daily Amount.

The GDA for saturates for an adult consuming 2000 calories per day is 20 g.

The GDA for saturates for an adult consuming 1700 calories per day is 17 g.

IMPORTANT NOTE: Your saturated fat GDA is *part of* your overall fat GDA. Don't make the mistake of thinking that you can add both totals together and eat more fat.

All these foods are high in saturated fat:

► meat products, meat pies, sausages
► hard cheese
► butter and lard
► pastry
► cakes and biscuits
► cream, soured cream and crème fraîche
► coconut oil, coconut cream and palm oil

Trans fats

Trans fats have a similar effect on blood cholesterol to saturated fats: they raise the type of cholesterol in the blood that increases the risk of heart disease. Trans fats are formed when liquid vegetable oils are turned into solid fats through the process of hydrogenation. In the UK, the use of hydrogenated vegetable oils has been greatly reduced over the past few years and this has helped reduce the amount of trans fats in many foods.

These changes mean that most people in the UK no longer eat large amounts of trans fats. On average we consume about half the recommended maximum – which is good news for our health. Most people eat a lot more saturated fat than trans fats, which is why GDAs focus on saturated fat. Trans fats don't need to be labelled separately under European law, so it's not so easy to see at a glance which foods contain them.

The most common foods containing trans fats are:

► bought biscuits and cakes
► fast food
► ready-made pastry
► some margarines

These sorts of food are usually high in saturated fat, sugar or salt as well, so if you are trying to eat a healthy diet, you'll be keeping these to a minimum anyway. Trans fats are also found naturally at very low levels in foods such as dairy products, beef and lamb, but not at a level you need to worry about.

Unsaturated fats

Unsaturated fats, which include polyunsaturated fats like sunflower oil and monounsaturated fats like olive oil, are a healthier choice than saturated or trans fats. It's important to remember, though, that unsaturated fats contain the same number of calories as the less healthy saturated and trans fats.

Unsaturated fats can contribute to reducing cholesterol levels and provide us with the essential fatty acids that our body needs. They include the unsaturated fats like omega-3 fatty acids found in oily fish, which may help protect against heart disease. All unsaturated fats are included in the GDAs and on GDA labels for total fat.

The following foods are all high in unsaturated fat:

▶ oily fish
▶ avocados
▶ nuts and seeds
▶ sunflower, rapeseed and olive oil and spreads (use sunflower and rapeseed oil for cooking and keep olive oil for salad dressings)

Some unsaturated fats, such as olive oil, change their chemical structure when they're heated and lose some of their potential health benefits.

Try to have unsaturated fat rather than saturated fat in your diet. This means you could choose:

▶ oily fish instead of sausages or a meat pie
▶ unsaturated oils such as sunflower or rapeseed when cooking, instead of butter, lard and ghee

- olive oil-based vinaigrette for salad dressings instead of creamy dressings like Blue Cheese, Thousand Island or Caesar dressing
- unsalted nuts rather than a biscuit when snacking
- mashed potato made with olive oil and garlic instead of butter and milk
- a spread that's high in unsaturated fat instead of butter
- 1% fat skimmed milk, instead of whole or semi-skimmed milk, if you drink more than half a litre (1 pint) per day.

Watch your fat levels

Any product using GDA labels will tell you how much total fat and saturated fat the food contains, but when there aren't GDA labels you'll still see figures for the total fat content on most foods, if you check the nutrition panel on the back of the pack. Some foods will also give figures for saturated fat, or 'saturates'. Compare the labels of different food products and choose those with less fat and less saturated fat. If there's no GDA label, use the following as a guide to work out if a food is high or low in fat.

Total fat – what's high and what's low?
High   20 g total fat or more per 100 g
Medium   3 g to 20g total fat per 100 g
Low   3 g total fat or less per 100 g

Saturated fat – what's high and what's low?
High   5 g saturates or more per 100 g
Medium   1.5 g to 5 g saturates per 100 g
Low   1.5 g saturates or less per 100 g

Tips for cutting down on your fat intake

Here are some practical suggestions to help you cut down on fat, especially saturated fat:

▶ Choose lean cuts of meat and trim off any visible fat.

▶ Grill, bake, poach or steam rather than frying and roasting so you don't need to add any extra fat.

▶ If you do choose to eat something high in fat such as a meat pie, pick something low in fat to go with it to make the whole meal lower in fat. For example, you could have a baked potato instead of chips.

▶ When you're choosing a ready meal or buying another food product, CHECK and COMPARE the labels so you can CHOOSE those with less total fat or less saturated fat.

▶ Put extra vegetables, beans or lentils and less meat in your casseroles and stews.

▶ Measure oil for cooking with teaspoons rather than pouring it straight from a container.

▶ Choose pies that have only one crust rather than two – either a lid or a base – because pastry is very high in fat. Avoid eating the crust on a pasty for the same reason.

▶ When you're making sandwiches, try not to use any butter or spread if the filling is moist enough. When you do use margarine or butter, opt for a reduced-fat variety and choose one that's soft, rather than using it straight from the fridge, so it's easier to spread thinly.

▶ Choose lower-fat versions of dairy foods whenever you can, such as semi-skimmed or skimmed milk, reduced-fat yoghurt, lower-fat cheese or very strong-tasting cheese, so you don't need to use as much.

▶ Instead of using cream or soured cream in recipes, try low or reduced fat yoghurt or fromage frais instead.

What about omega-3s?

Oily fish is the best source of omega-3 fatty acids. These fatty acids have been shown to help protect against coronary heart disease. There has also been some inconclusive research suggesting other health benefits for omega-3 fatty acids, including their effect on children's brain development. (For more information, see The British Dietetic Association website: www.bda.uk.com where you will find the latest food facts and useful download.) The general advice is that most of us should aim to include more fish and omega-3s in our diets.

Some omega-3 fatty acids are found in certain vegetable oils, such as linseed walnut, soya and rapeseed. These aren't quite the same type of fatty acids as those found in fish, but are a useful alternative for people following a vegetarian diet. We should all try to eat two portions of fish a week. One portion of white fish and one portion of oily fish is an excellent target to aim for.

► White fish include plaice, halibut, skate, cod and haddock
► Oily fish include salmon, fresh tuna, trout, sardines, pilchards and mackerel

"I knew that eating too much saturated fat wasn't good for my heart, but I hadn't realised that my waist measurement indicated a risk factor. Now, after following the GDA Diet for six months, I've lost three inches from my waist and I know which foods have a lot of saturates in them. It's been a win–win situation!"
John C, Bedfordshire

SALT

We need to be wary of salt. Many of us are regularly eating around 9.5 g of salt a day – which is 50% more than our adult GDA of 6 g per day. Too much salt in our diet has been linked to problems such as high blood pressure and heart disease, so a diet that stays within the Guideline Daily Amount for salt is something we should all be aiming for, whether we're trying to lose weight or not.

> The GDA for salt for an average adult is 6 g, whatever their calorie intake.

Sodium

The white stuff we sprinkle on our chips is known to most of us as table salt, but when it comes to food labels salt will often be shown using its chemical name: Sodium Chloride. Sodium is an essential mineral required by the body. One of its functions is to help balance the levels of fluid in the body, which helps to maintain normal blood pressure and keep nerves and muscles working properly. However, an excessive intake of sodium may cause problems for some people and a wealth of evidence links sodium intake with high blood pressure (hypertension).

The UK Government's Scientific Advisory Committee on Nutrition (SACN) has set targets for salt intake reduction because there is evidence that reducing sodium in the diet helps lower blood pressure in people with both high and normal blood pressure. Of course, several other factors have an important role in controlling blood pressure too, such as your body weight, level of daily activity and the amount of alcohol you drink.

Confusing labelling

Most packaged food products carry a nutrition label on the back of the pack that, in line with current legislation, states the sodium content rather than the salt content – which isn't really that helpful. To work out the equivalent amount of salt, multiply the sodium value by 2.5 (e.g. 1.2g sodium is equivalent to 3.0g salt). Luckily, you don't have to worry about this when it come to GDA labels. The GDA label shows the salt level and has done all the maths for you. You only need to be aware of the sodium/salt conundrum if you're using the back-of-pack information to check, compare and choose.

Some packs also provide a 'salt equivalent' figure based on this calculation, as shown in this example.

NUTRITIONAL INFORMATION for chicken and vegetable bake		
Typical values	per 100g	per 350g pack
Energy – kJ	480kJ	1680kJ
- kcal	115kcal	405kcal
Protein	9.5g	33.3g
Carbohydrate	8.6g	30.1g
of which sugars	3.5g	12.3g
Fat	4.6g	16.1g
of which saturates	2.0g	7.0g
Fibre	1.5g	5.3g
Sodium*	0.3g	1.1g
*Equivalent as salt	0.8g	2.8g

Sodium – what's high or low?

The Food Standards Agency (FSA) recommends the following guidelines:

A lot   0.5g sodium or more per 100g of food
A little   0.1g sodium or less per 100g of food

However, take account of the portion size of the food you eat to help gauge the amount of sodium. For example, certain foods, such as yeast extracts, are relatively high in sodium at 45g per 100g, but are eaten in very small quantities as an average serving is 4g, which means you'd actually be eating 1.8g per serving.

Tips for cutting down on your salt intake

Shopping

▶ Check the nutrition labels to keep track of your salt and sodium intake.

▶ Look for 'reduced salt' or 'reduced sodium' advice on packs. These foods should be at least 25% lower in salt than the standard product. Opt for 'reduced-salt' versions of foods whenever possible, including bread, baked beans, crisps, biscuits, butter, fat spreads, soups, gravy granules, crackers and ready meals.

▶ Choose canned vegetables marked 'no added salt' and products such as tuna that are canned in water rather than brine.

▶ Try using 'low-sodium' salt substitutes for use in cooking and at the table (but don't use these if you have kidney problems).

▶ Cut down on inherently salty foods: cured meat, cheese, smoked meat and fish, olives, anchovies and soy sauce.

Cooking

▶ Aim to reduce the amount of salt used in cooking – do this gradually, as your tastebuds may take time to adjust.

▶ If a recipe tells you to reduce the volume of a stock, add the seasoning after the 'reducing' stage, rather than before.

▶ Experiment! We all want tasty food, so replace salt with other flavours. Try different herbs such as basil, chives, lemon grass, rosemary or coriander, and spices such as chilli, ginger, garlic or cumin.

▶ Taste your food before adding salt at the table, and then take just a little if needed.

Eating out

▶ When your food arrives, taste it before adding salt. If you feel more salt is needed, add only a little.

▶ Moderate the amount of sauces you add, such as soy sauce, as they can be high in salt.

You don't have to stop eating foods that are higher in salt, as all foods can fit into a healthy balanced diet. However, if you eat several high-salt foods, cut back on the salt in other foods at other times to maintain a balance. Remember that the daily target intake of 6g salt (2.4g sodium) for adults is a maximum.

If you have hypertension or another medical condition you may need to follow a stricter diet plan – if in doubt, always check with your doctor.

"We have a family history of stroke, so I've always tried to look after myself and eat well. GDAs have really opened my eyes to where the salt is in my food. It's great to have extra reassurance that I'm eating the right foods."
Audrey D, Northamptonshire

THE FOOD INDUSTRY

It's a popular sport in our media to attack the food industry as being responsible for the UK's obesity and weight 'epidemic'. It has also been under attack for adding salt to our food. The truth is that the blame for the state of our nation's health cannot ever be laid at one group's door – we all have a part to play. It's only fair that I try to put the record straight and let you see some of the big steps the food industry is taking to make our food better for us. The reductions achieved in the amount of salt added to our food are a shining example!

▶ Bread – sodium levels have reduced by about 25% since the late 1980s, and recently by a further 5% in sliced bread.
▶ Breakfast cereals – manufacturers achieved a 33% reduction in sodium between 1998 and 2005.

- ▶ Savoury snacks – sodium levels have reduced significantly in the past decade. Potato crisps are now 25% lower in sodium.
- ▶ Soups and cook-in sauces – manufacturers have achieved a 25% reduction in sodium levels in soups and a 29% reduction in cook-in sauces since 2003.
- ▶ Cakes – reductions of up to 40% have been achieved in the sodium content some of most popular brands of cakes and mince pies.
- ▶ Biscuits – reductions of up to 20% have been achieved in the sodium content of some of the most popular brands of biscuits.

GDA DIET SUCCESS SECRETS

1 Enjoy the fact that as well as helping you save calories, GDAs are helping you to stay within the recommended maximum amounts of total fat, saturates, sugar and salt you need to be healthy.

2 By controlling your weight you are reducing your risk of coronary heart disease, diabetes and some cancers.

3 If a product doesn't have a GDA label on the front, you can still use the nutritional information on the back to help you keep a track of what's inside your food.

6 IT'S ALL IN THE PLANNING

The GDA Diet is designed to be very flexible. There's a plan for busy people who just don't have the time or the inclination for cooking; a vegetarian plan for people who don't want to eat meat; and a budget plan for people who are watching the pennies as well as their waistline. You can just opt in and out of whichever plan suits you.

If you know you're pretty constant in your approach to food or you like the idea of a prescriptive eating plan, then pick a plan and follow it to the letter for a week to get into the swing of things. The scientific research behind GDAs tells me that the principles of the diet can be adapted to suit *everyone*. All I've done is taken those principles and made them work in a flexible format, to suit as many people as possible. It's fine to choose a breakfast from the vegetarian plan, a lunch from the plan for busy people and have a budget dinner in the evening, if you want to; but make sure you stick to either the 2000-calorie plans or the 1700-calorie plans.

I have quite deliberately included a lot of convenience meals and snacks in all of the plans because I really want you to see how easy it is to follow the GDA Diet. However, if you're like me, you probably use a mixture of meals cooked from scratch and convenience food throughout the week; and that's OK too. If you decide you want to make your own Shepherd's Pie or Spaghetti Bolognese go right ahead, but have a look at my healthy cooking tips on page 162 to help keep your home-cooked dishes GDA friendly.

There is no restrictive 'start-up' phase of the GDA Diet to leave you feeling hungry, deprived or miserable. These plans have been designed to give you results that are nutritionally balanced, so that once you start you can just keep on going.

Before you start, you first need to choose the calorie allowance that best suits your weight-loss needs.

CHOOSING THE RIGHT GDA DIET PLAN

The GDAs you see on the front of food packs are set for both men and women and are a general guide for healthy eating rather than weight loss. However, when regular GDAs are combined with some physical activity they become the perfect weight-loss plan, and are suitable for those with a significant amount of weight to lose.

Make sure you're being honest with yourself when you choose your calorie allowance. Don't be tempted to opt for the lower-calorie plan if you have more than 13 kg (2 stone) to lose. You won't get faster results. Instead, the likelihood is that if the plan has too few calories for you, you'll get too hungry and give up. That would just be another trip around the diet cycle, so **please read the next couple of sections to choose the right plan.**

Weight loss GDAs for men and for women who need to lose more than 13 kg (2 stone)

The GDA values used as a basis for the labels you see on the front of over 20,000 food packs are perfect for you. If you follow the 20:30:30:20 guide I talked about in Chapter 3 you'll be consuming around 2000 calories a day, as well as the right amount of fat, saturates and sugar and salt to be healthy. With a fairly modest amount of activity each day (30–40 minutes), you should easily be able to lose a safe, steady and maintainable amount of weight (around 1–2 lb or ½–1 kg) per week.

Your GDA for calories is 2000, your total GDA for fat is 70 g, and for saturates it's 20 g. Your GDA for sugar is 90 g and for salt it's 6 g.

That breaks down into 20:30:30:20 as follows:

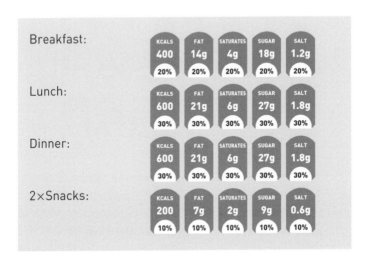

Breakfast:

KCALS	FAT	SATURATES	SUGAR	SALT
400	14g	4g	18g	1.2g
20%	20%	20%	20%	20%

Lunch:

KCALS	FAT	SATURATES	SUGAR	SALT
600	21g	6g	27g	1.8g
30%	30%	30%	30%	30%

Dinner:

KCALS	FAT	SATURATES	SUGAR	SALT
600	21g	6g	27g	1.8g
30%	30%	30%	30%	30%

2×Snacks:

KCALS	FAT	SATURATES	SUGAR	SALT
200	7g	2g	9g	0.6g
10%	10%	10%	10%	10%

I have also created an adaptation of the standard GDAs with a calorie allowance of 1700 (instead of 2000) for women with only a small amount of weight to lose (most men need more than this level of calories).

Weight loss GDAs for women who need to lose less than 13 kg (2 stone)

Your GDA for calories is 1700, your total GDA for fat is 60 g and for saturates it's 17 g. Your GDA for sugar is 76.5 g and for salt it's 6 g

That breaks down into 20:30:30:20 as follows:

Breakfast:

KCALS	FAT	SATURATES	SUGAR	SALT
340	12g	3.4g	15.3g	1.2g
20%	20%	20%	20%	20%

Lunch:

KCALS	FAT	SATURATES	SUGAR	SALT
510	18g	5.1g	22.95g	1.8g
30%	30%	30%	30%	30%

Dinner:

KCALS	FAT	SATURATES	SUGAR	SALT
510	18g	5.1g	22.95g	1.8g
30%	30%	30%	30%	30%

2×Snack:

KCALS	FAT	SATURATES	SUGAR	SALT
170	6g	1.7g	7.6g	0.6g
10%	10%	10%	10%	10%

Remember, I don't want you to get too worried about all these numbers. You don't need to be too exact about this – think of it as a rough guide. If you go over target on a nutrient such as fat at one meal, then just choose a lower-fat option at another. I usually recommend that snacks are divided into two: one in the morning (10%) and one mid-afternoon (10%).

P IS FOR PLANNING SUCCESS

Planning is vital. To help you to remember to plan, think about, and repeat to yourself, the 4Ps:

Proper
Planning
Produces
Permanent weight management

It's true – I promise you!

Let's face it, you're about to try to change something you've done the same way every single day of your life: the way you eat. If you just 'jump in' without giving the process deeper thought, isn't it likely that you're going to make a mistake or forget something? That's not about a lack of willpower, it's human nature!

When I look back at my clients' past dieting disasters, one of the biggest causes of 'failure' is usually that there was no planning. They just jumped right in. Think about it, you already have great planning skills: perhaps you run a house, or have a busy job or plan the kids' schedule. You wouldn't head off on a journey without knowing where you were going, and you would probably take a map too (or use sat nav!) to keep you on the right road. There's no greater journey than the path back to good health, so it makes sense to decide the best route to your weight-loss destination by planning your food shopping and menu.

Planning doesn't need to become a military exercise, but at least make sure you know what you're going to eat for the next few days and whether those recipes are going to work with your schedule.

The layout of the eating plans and food lists has been designed to make food planning as easy and as flexible as possible. But – like any other tool – these are only helpful if you use them properly. The plans are there as a guide to get you started.

I have divided the plans into separate ones to suit busy people, vegetarians and people on a budget to illustrate to you how GDAs really can work for *everyone* who wants to eat well and control their weight. Only use the plans in a prescriptive way (eat this on Monday and that on Tuesday) if that's what's going to suit *you*. If you would prefer to mix the plans up and add in your own home-cooked dishes, that's OK too – but remember to use *either* the 2000-calorie plan or the 1700-calorie plan. Don't mix these. Also, use my cooking tips on page 171 to make sure your home-cooked meals keep you on the right side of the GDA tracks.

There are literally tens of thousands of foods to choose from that have GDA labels. So once you're comfortable using GDAs, feel free to go beyond the foods in my eating plans and food lists and start making your own plans.

Remember: GDA labels are just a tool to tell you what's inside your food. *You* are the boss, not the GDAs!

This is how I suggest you plan for your first week. Take a quiet half hour or so the week before you want to start. Sit down with this book and look at the eating plans. Then check your diary and see what the week ahead is like. Ask yourself these important questions:

- ▶ Will I be eating at home every night?
- ▶ What foods will I have to buy to make sure I keep on track this week?
- ▶ Can I take my lunch with me to work?
- ▶ What snacks will I be eating?
- ▶ Do I need to remind myself to take snacks with me so I don't get tempted to buy foods I'm trying to avoid when I get peckish?

Make your eating plan fit in with your schedule, not the other way around!

1 Choose your meals and snacks from your preferred diet plan – but make sure they fit in with your weekly schedule.

2 Then look at the fast-and-easy recipes and see what you need to stock up on.

3 Write a list of everything you need – and that's your personal weekly shopping list done.

Proper planning means you're off to the perfect start. If you've chosen some of the ready meals or other convenience foods and snacks I mention in the plans, just check the products available in your usual supermarket to make sure they meet the same percentage of GDAs.

APPLYING THE 20:30:30:20 RULE TO THE 2000-CALORIE PLAN

In Chapter 3 I introduced the 20:30:30:20 rule as the ideal way to keep track of the amounts you're eating.

20:30:30:20 keeps you on track from morning to night.

The table below shows you the figures for all the GDA nutrients using the 20:30:30:20 rule. The calories are shown in **bold.**

Your targets are 400 calories for breakfast, 600 calories at lunch, 600 calories at dinner and two snacks of around 200 calories each during the day. Total calories 2000.

	Calories	Sugar	Fat	Saturated fats	Salt
Total for the day	**2000**	90 g	70 g	20 g	6 g
Breakfast 20%	**400**	18 g	14 g	4 g	1.2 g
Lunch 30%	**600**	27 g	21 g	6 g	1.8 g
Dinner 30%	**600**	27 g	21 g	6 g	1.8 g
Snack×2 10% each	**200**	9 g	7 g	2 g	0.6 g

The GDA Diet meal plans (see Chapter 8) are there to help you get the hang of the 20:30:30:20 routine. Each meal has just about the right amount of calories for each breakfast, lunch, dinner and snack. That's right – snack! You can snack on the GDA Diet, in fact I positively encourage you to, because people who are savvy snackers are less likely to graze on fatty, sugary foods – and that helps them to keep in shape.

Sample day from the 2000-calorie meal plans

Breakfast	Snack	Lunch	Snack	Dinner
CALORIES 400 20%	**CALORIES 200** 10%	**CALORIES 600** 30%	**CALORIES 200** 10%	**CALORIES 600** 30%
150g melon 1 Toasted English muffin 1 slice wholemeal toast with 3 tsp reduced-fat spread and 3 tsp jam	5 water biscuits 3 tsp low-fat soft cheese Handful grapes	Salmon and cucumber sandwich Toasted tea cake 1 tsp reduced-fat spread 150ml orange juice	1 banana 1 tbsp low-fat yogurt 1 tbsp no-added-sugar muesli	Chicken and broccoli pie with carrots and sweetcorn Stewed apple and 3 tbsp custard made with skimmed milk

I have designed the GDA Diet so that you achieve your daily requirement nutritional. As well as keeping an eye on the amount of fat, sugar and salt in the meal plans, there are also plenty of fruit and vegetables, dairy foods, grains and protein foods such as meats, fish, poultry, nuts, beans and pulses. That means your body will get everything it needs for a nutritionally balanced diet, without having too much of the things you don't need. Add a little activity into the mix and before you know it, you're losing weight!

APPLYING THE 20:30:30:20 RULE TO THE 1700-CALORIE PLAN

The table below shows you the figures for all the GDA nutrients using the 20:30:30:20 rule, with the calories shown in **bold.**

Your targets are 340 calories for breakfast, 510 calories at lunch, 510 calories at dinner, and two snacks of 170 calories each. Total calories 1700.

	Calories	Sugar	Fat	Saturated fats	Salt
GDA for the day	1700	76.5g	60g	17g	6g
Breakfast 20%	340	15.3g	12g	3.4g	1.2g
Lunch 30%	510	22.95g	18g	5.1g	1.8g
Dinner 30%	510	22.95g	18g	5.1g	1.8g
Snack×2 10% each	170	7.65g	6g	1.7g	0.6g

The meal plans for the 1700-calorie GDA Diet (see chapter 8) are there to help you get the hang of the 20:30:30:20 rule. I have calculated the GDAs for you for each meal. Everyone has the right level of calories and nutrients per breakfast, lunch, dinner and snack to total 1700 calories for the day.

Sample day from the 1700-calorie meal plans

Breakfast	**Snack**	**Lunch**	**Snack**	**Dinner**
CALORIES 340 20%	CALORIES 170 10%	CALORIES 510 30%	CALORIES 170 10%	CALORIES 510 36%
125ml fruit juice 2 slices wholegrain toast with 2 tsp reduced-fat spread and 2 tsp jam	4 small water biscuits 2 tsp low-fat soft cheese Apple	Salmon and cucumber sandwich Cereal and dried fruit bar	125g pot probiotic yogurt Handful grapes	Chicken and broccoli pie with 2 portions vegetables Handful raspberries with small meringue nest/shell 1 tbsp low-fat yogurt

You'll notice from this sample menu that the 1700-calorie meal plans are very similar to the 2000-calorie plans. You may just have a slightly smaller portion, or there may be a change to one part of your meal that will make the extra calorie, fat or sugar savings you need. So that you don't waste food, I've tried to make sure that your calorie savings come from snacks and desserts rather than the main meals. For example, if you buy a pie, such as the chicken and broccoli pie listed here, you can have the same portion size as someone on the 2000-calorie plan, safe in the knowledge that you've saved 300 calories during the day by eating smaller snacks and choosing a lower-calorie dessert.

Once you've reached your target weight, you shouldn't keep on dieting. Instead, you need to maintain, rather than continue to lose weight. You can simply increase your target calorie intake to 2000 calories per day.

I have not picked specific brands for the eating plans deliberately, because we all shop in different places, but where, for instance, I've suggested lasagne for dinner or cereal for breakfast, remember to refer to the 20:30:30:20 GDA amounts when deciding which brand to opt for.

Where I have suggested a ready meal or a generic product like a breakfast cereal, I have looked at all the major supermarkets' own brands and the large, popular brands to make sure that the foods and products are widely available wherever you live, and that they all have similar GDA profiles to those listed in my GDA diet eating plans. So I feel confident that you'll be able to buy foods with similar GDA values to those in the plans wherever you shop.

20:30:30:20 helps you spread your GDAs throughout the day

GDAs at breakfast	20% of total
GDAs at lunch	30% of total
GDAs at dinner	30% of total
GDAs for two snacks	20% of total
Total GDAs for day	100%

I want you to get used to using the GDAs as soon as possible, and grocery shopping is the best way to get you into the habit of reading GDA labels and using them to CHECK, COMPARE and CHOOSE your meals. After a week or two of doing this you'll get quicker and quicker at it and it will begin to feel like second nature. Making sure that you have everything you need in the house before you start a new week on the diet is one of the most effective ways of successfully beating your old diet cycle.

YOU NEVER HAVE TO BE BORED

There's absolutely no reason for you to get bored or hungry on the GDA Diet. There are thousands of products out there with GDA labels on the front of the pack, and many thousands more showing the GDA values on the back of the pack, so there's never any need to get into a dull, repetitive food routine. If you tend to buy the same foods each week, then try some new options to fit into your plan.

As long as you stay close the 20:30:30:20 GDA guidelines, you'll be just fine.

If you find you're hungry, then have another look at your chosen GDA diet plan and make sure you're following the guidelines and eating all the meals and snacks. Snacking is an essential part of the GDA Diet and it's far better to pre-empt hunger than to wait until you're so hungry that you grab anything in sight! If you snack consciously and regularly and don't allow yourself to get too ravenous, you're far more likely to choose healthy foods.

Keep an eye on the GDA Diet *success secrets* at the end of each chapter. They will remind you of all the most important points. Have a look at the GDA Diet website (www.GDAdiet.com) for lots of tips and expert advice too.

EATING OUT

The problem with being on a diet is that having a night out can cause panic and lead to diet sabotage. There's no need to worry. Try to find out in advance what type of restaurant you'll be going to, and use some of the tips below to help you stay in the driving seat:

► Make sure you eat regularly throughout the day. If you're ravenous by the time you go out for dinner, it will be really difficult to make any healthy choices.

► Enjoy going out! It's rare that food is the only focal point – friends, family and fun are important too. Love the food and focus on the company.

► See if the restaurant has a website so you can have a look at the menu before you go. You can then choose in advance, without the pressure of a waiter breathing down your neck.

► Choose fruit- or salad-based starters and ask for dressing on the side. Clear soups are a great choice too.

► Waiters are so used to fussy eaters or special dietary needs these days that asking for salad instead of chips, sauces on the side or a fruit-based dessert won't even cause a raised eyebrow.

- Starters are often a good source of healthy ingredients: pulses, fish and vegetables. So if the main courses are looking unpromising, have two starters instead. It's amazing how filling two starters can be.
- Dessert is a tricky option to resist, especially at a dinner party. Have a small taster if you really feel you can't refuse, or wait for cheese if that's on offer. The best choices will be strawberries, fruit salad, a small portion of cheese with fruit or some plain ice cream.
- Alcoholic drinks in all forms make weak-willed folk out of all of us! So take it easy. Every time you have a drink, you're delaying your weight loss. You're also far more likely to say 'oh, go on then' as the cream or calorie-laden dessert comes round. If you are drinking, match your alcoholic drink with a glass of water. You will end up drinking less alcohol and feel a whole lot better in the morning.
- Hardest of all will be the dinner party when there's no way of choosing the food you end up with on your plate. Eat smaller amounts of foods you know will be high in fat and sugar (the main calorie culprits) and fill up on veggies and salad. That way you can still be polite and feel virtuous. Remember, it's only one meal, so if you're not perfect it's not the end of the world.
- In reality, we're all going to be faced with no-GDA moments. When this happens, don't panic. Enjoy the food and watch your portion sizes. Try to make sure that no more than a quarter of what's on your plate is made up of foods that are bad for your diet (e.g. pastry, puddings, creamy sauces, fatty meats, fried foods, creamy salad dressings and so on). Make sure that the majority of your food includes undressed salads, vegetables, fruit, grilled meats, fish and poultry, pasta with tomato-based sauces, boiled rice, plain potatoes (not roasted or mashed potatoes) and so on.

- Buffets are easy once you've got your head around GDA quantities. Salads, fish, meat, a few new potatoes or some crusty bread are all OK. Stay away from pastry and mayonnaise-laden sandwiches and creamy puddings.
- Not all 'fast food' is bad these days; thankfully many fast food restaurants are actively adapting their offerings to incorporate GDA labels. Many have very informative websites telling you about the nutritional values of their meals, so when you have a few minutes check out your favourites and see how they stack up GDA-wise.
- If you're just going out for drinks, then eat a sensible, balanced GDA meal before you go and set a limit on the number of drinks you have during the evening.

"As soon as I started getting a bit more organised with my food the weight started to come off. It had never occurred to me that it was so important. Now I never find myself diving into the biscuit barrel because I just don't buy them!"
Melanie W., Surrey

GDA DIET SUCCESS SECRETS

1 Don't dwell on any past dieting disappointments. Instead, reflect on and understand what went wrong in the past and learn from it.

2 Plan ahead. Creating menus and shopping lists will help to keep you in the diet driving seat.

3 You don't need to go hungry. The GDA Diet gives you three meals a day plus two snacks – so eat regularly. If you get too hungry you're far more likely to make a mistake.

4 Socialise with confidence. Check ahead for restaurant menus and use the tips on page 67 to help you cope with dinner parties.

7 GOAL SETTING AND GETTING STARTED

We talked in Chapter 6 about the importance of planning ahead before you start your diet. An important part of planning is deciding what it is you actually want to achieve. You might be thinking at this point, 'It's obvious – if I'm reading a diet book, I just want to lose weight!'

However, there are plenty of other benefits that would come your way as you lose weight. Setting goals for these outcomes too is a great way to keep on track if you feel yourself being tempted to stray off the healthy path.

For example, you might want to:

▶ feel more confident
▶ be able to buy clothes more easily
▶ lower your risk of heart disease, diabetes, cancer or other diseases
▶ improve your level of fitness
▶ increase your energy levels

Or your goal might be as simple as wanting to get back into that dress or the suit you haven't been able to wear for ages.

GOAL SETTING
Whatever you want for yourself, the art of goal setting is to keep your goals 'real' and achievable. Setting performance measures or milestones as personal markers along the way will help you to know – and see and feel – that you're

heading in the right direction while on your journey. Don't be tempted to set yourself a huge goal that feels so insurmountable that you may not take the first step. Instead, set yourself small, steady, manageable steps that are easy to make and will gradually build into a permanent change in lifestyle. Knowing you're being successful as you continue along on your journey will help to keep you focused and motivated.

I've been very careful throughout the book to keep my promises realistic and achievable and I really want to encourage you to do the same with your expectations of yourself. If you set unrealistic, unachievable goals, you also set yourself up for disappointment and failure – and most of us know what that feels like from our past experiences, don't we?

THE REALITY OF WEIGHT LOSS

Weight loss is never consistent. Nobody loses the same amount of weight every week, and I can promise you that if we were to put 100 people on the same diet and followed them for a year, none of them would lose weight every single week. So, rather than focusing on your weekly weight loss, the way I prefer to measure success is to look at monthly weight loss. By taking three or four weight measurements during the month and then averaging them at the end of a full month, you will get a much more accurate picture of what's going on. This method evens out the results of those weeks where weight loss is disappointing with those where it all seems to be going so well. Monthly weight figures 'keep it real' and help prevent the emotional highs and lows that lead to false expectations or disappointments.

The one thing I would ask is that you don't get into the habit of weighing yourself every day or, even worse, more than once a day. Use the same scales, on the same day, at about the same time of day once a week. We can weigh up to 4 pounds heavier from one end of the day to the next just because we're holding more fluid, so weighing yourself at the same time of day is important.

> I've seen so many of my clients ride an emotional roller-coaster of misery and ecstasy as they jump on and off the scales two or three times a day. Their mood is driven by the scales telling them about their state of hydration, *not* about how much fat they're carrying. This is, of course, a complete waste of emotional energy and can be very destructive.

If you think you're likely to be tempted to weigh yourself more than once a week, then I would suggest you move your scales so you have to dig them out of the wardrobe or the garage to use them. Don't keep the scales right under your nose in the bathroom. They'll soon start calling you to jump on every time you're in there – and you'll get a false idea of your progress.

It will also help you to achieve your goals if you set yourself long-term targets. There are literally hundreds of ways to decide these. I'll look at a few of the most important in the next section.

> A once-a-week weigh-in, at the same time of day and using the same equipment, is one of my golden rules. But remember – the once-a-month average is the figure to pay attention to.

WEIGHT LOSS FOR HEALTH

If you're quite overweight – let's say your Body Mass Index (BMI) is over 30 – and you're dieting for health reasons, then setting a goal to reach a BMI of 20 might not be immediately realistic. If your goal seems too far away, it won't be helpful in keeping you motivated. Instead, aim first of all to reduce your weight by 10 per cent. (For information about how to calculate your BMI, see page 33.)

How does this work? Let's say you currently weigh 101 kg (i.e. 16 stone or 224 lb): a 10 per cent weight reduction would be 10 kg (i.e. 1½ stone or 22½ lb). Once you've reached this target, you simply set your next target of 10 per cent and carry on. Breaking weight-loss goals into small, achievable targets is much more manageable than having a start point and one long-term end point.

The 10 per cent target is very significant. Good-quality studies (see www.sign.ac.uk/) have shown that reducing your weight by as little as 10 per cent significantly reduces your risk of heart disease, diabetes, high blood pressure, high cholesterol and some cancers. It's not a result to be sniffed at. Once you get to 10 per cent, aim for the next 10 per cent and so on – the health benefits just keep on coming.

GETTING YOUR MEASURE

Fat carried around the tummy or abdomen is a key indicator for an increased risk of heart disease and diabetes, so aiming to reduce your waist to a circumference that reduces health risks is a fantastic goal.

	Increased risk	Substantial risk
	Waist circumference	*Waist circumference*
Men	94 cm (37 in) or more	102 cm (40 in) or more
Women	80 cm (32 in) or more	88 cm (35 in) or more

I've included a measurement chart for you to complete. This will be particularly useful if you plan to continue your diet for a few weeks. You will feel more motivated to continue if you can see that your progress is moving in the right direction.

	Today	*+4 wks*	*+4 wks*	*+4 wks*	*+4 wks*	*+4 wks*	*Target*
Bust							
Waist							
Hips							
Weight							
BMI							
Clothes size							

If you're not sure how to take accurate measurements then have a look at my tips on page 35.

As far as other measures of success go, the key is to record where you are right now, before you start the diet, and then to make regular appointments with yourself to revisit your list and review your progress. Ask yourself about your feelings, emotions, levels of confidence and other weight-connected issues. There's much more to be gained from weight management than what the scales tell you. You can score these feelings and emotions in a variety of ways. Words are one good way, but if you find that difficult try using a scale of 1–10.

The Feelings Table

Imagine a scale from 1 to 10, where 1 represents the *least* confident or optimistic you could feel, and 10 represents the *most* confident or optimistic you could feel.

Ask yourself each week: on a scale of 1 to 10, how do I feel today?

Give yourself a score from 1–10 for all the categories on the feelings table and revisit the table every week as your diet progresses. Add further categories for other factors that are important to you.

Feelings table
Keep a record of how you feel here: 1 = lowest, 10 = highest

	Example	Week 1
Confidence	$\frac{4}{10}$	I'm still using the GDA eating plans, but beginning to be able to check, compare and choose foods for myself
Optimism	$\frac{9}{10}$	I'm really beginning to feel the benefit of eating well – I'm sure I can keep going
Planning	$\frac{8}{10}$	My shopping list for the week takes me about 10 minutes to write
Fitness	$\frac{3}{10}$	I'm still a bit puffed after my daily walk but it's slowly getting easier.
Body shape	$\frac{4}{10}$	Can fasten jeans – but not comfortable
Weight	$\frac{1}{10}$	11st 8lb (73kg)

Recording things other than your weight and physical measurements is motivating and an important factor to keep you going. It might seem a strange process to start with, but the more you do it, and the more honest you can be, the easier it will become.

"Losing the 2 stone I'd been carrying around with me for years has completely turned my life around. I hadn't realised the effect my weight was having on my self-esteem, but now I do things I'd never have dreamt of last year – I've even signed up to do a parachute jump."
Michael L, Sheffield

CALLING ALL SUPPORTERS

Before you start the GDA Diet, think about previous diets when you've been successful. Did you diet alone or with friends? A lot of people find that if they buddy up with someone else it can be really helpful. Others find that they just like to go it alone. There isn't a right or a wrong approach, but it's well worth thinking about what will suit you best. Is there someone who you think it would be good to diet with?

If you are going to diet with other people, choose your partnerships carefully. There are diet saboteurs out there who can subconsciously spoil your plan by encouraging you to take a short cut here or there. Make sure that the person you choose is really committed and is of a similar mindset to you.

Support can come in many guises when we diet, it's usually meant to be helpful but sometimes people just don't support us in the best way. Nagging, bullying and humiliation are thoroughly unhelpful and a sure-fire way to make you rebel and abandon your diet. Decide first whether you want to tell people you're trying to lose weight. For some people, telling their loved ones reinforces their commitment.

Choose your dieting friends wisely. Decide what they can best do to help you and ask them for what you need. If you don't want them to eat biscuits in front of you, ask them not to. If you want them to ask you how you're getting on once a week rather than every 5 minutes, or if you'd prefer them not to mention it at all, tell your friends your preference. Ask them to ask any questions they have in a way that doesn't sound accusing or patronising.

Decide on the kind of support you want and will respond best to and ask for it! If you prefer your support to come from people who are less involved with your day-to-day life, then there are some great supportive websites out there for people who are managing their weight, with interactive chat rooms and expert advice. One of my favourites is www.buddypower.co.uk. And of course, you can also join up to www.GDAdiet.com.

GDA DIET SUCCESS SECRETS

1 Set realistic, achievable goals and break them down into small, manageable steps.

2 Measure your success in as many ways as possible. There is a lot more to enjoy about being in control of your weight than the result on the scales.

3 Find the right kind of support from friends, relatives and websites. All are useful, but be sure to ask for the kind of support you need.

4 Remember: this isn't a quick-fix, crash diet. It's a sensible, healthy eating and activity plan for life!

PART III
THE GDA DIET

8 THE GDA DIET 7-DAY EATING PLANS

Every person who follows the GDA Diet will be different. You'll have different schedules, different family sizes, different tastes in food, and of course different cooking skills. It therefore makes sense that you will probably end up following slightly different GDA eating plans. The good news is the GDA Diet plans are flexible enough to allow exactly that.

The most important thing to do first is use the information on page 29 to work out whether you need to follow the 2000-calorie or 1700-calorie eating plan. This is the only part of the GDA Diet I ask you to stick to rigidly, as it will ensure that you lose weight at a maintainable rate and still get all the nutrients you need to be healthy. After that, it's your choices all the way.

Both the 2000-calorie and 1700-calorie plans include three weeks of day-by-day, mix-and-match menus:

▶ **The 7-day plan for busy people** contains mostly pre-prepared convenience foods that are available as popular, well-known and own brands in all major supermarkets around the UK.
▶ **The 7-day vegetarian plan** is full of tasty meals and snacks that are meat free.
▶ **The 7-day plan for people on a budget** gives you ideas to help you keep control of your purse strings as well as your weight.

Some people prefer to be shown exactly what to eat at each meal when they start a diet, and this can work very well. However, it's also useful to see how the basic framework of a diet can be adapted to suit your lifestyle. The good news is that as long as you stay within the 20:30:30:20 guidelines for your calorie allowance (2000 calories or 1700 calories), you can then adapt the 7-day eating plans in two ways.

Mix and match

You can either choose to follow one of the 7-day plans to the letter or mix and match all three plans according to your schedule. If you want to chop and change from one plan to another, just make sure that you have three meals and two snacks each day. You might choose a breakfast from the 7-day vegetarian plan, a lunch from the 7-day plan for busy people and your snacks and dinner from the 7-day plan for people on a budget (or of course, any combination of these). The choice is yours! As long as you stay with either 2000 calories or 1700 calories for the day you'll be on track. You can also use the additional meal and snack ideas (starting on page 143) as swaps for meals you don't fancy. Just make sure your swap fits in with the 20:30:30:20 guideline (see page 30).

Do it yourself

In a typical week, most people will eat a mix of pre-prepared ready meals and meals they've cooked from scratch. If you see a suggestion for a meal you would usually cook yourself, for instance sausage and mash or a pasta dish, then go ahead and use your favourite recipe – but adapt it by looking at my cooking tips on page 166, which are full of ways to reduce the high-fat, high-sugar, high-calorie dangers that are hidden within everyday recipes for familiar, family meals.

LET'S GET STARTED

If you are a man, or a woman with more than 13 kg (2 stone) to lose, you can use any of the 2000-calorie plans that follow. If you are a woman with less than 13 kg (2 stone) to lose, then any of the 1700-calorie plans will work for you. Men generally have higher calorie requirements than women, whether they need to lose weight or not, so I suggest most men follow the 2000-calorie plans.

It's not a good idea to mix the 1700-calorie plans with the 2000-calorie plans as they have been designed for different body weights and different levels of weight loss.

The foods in the plans can be bought at any supermarket and can be any brand. Each meal lists the GDA value using the 20:30:30:20 rule. For a list of retailers and manufacturers who are using GDA front-of-pack labels see page 225.

There are quick and easy recipes for some meals at the end of Chapter 8; all other meals are available as pre-prepared convenience foods. The plans are a tool to help you get used to reading the GDAs. If you feel confident enough to construct your own plan straight away – go for it.

You may notice that some of the plans exceed the daily GDA for sugar. This is because some of the sugar content derives naturally from the fruit or other carbohydrate ingredient content in the recipes and pre-prepared foods. These fruit sugars (fructose) and other natural occurring sugars are less of a concern than refined sugars because the foods in which they are found are also important sources of essential vitamins and minerals. So a little extra natural sugar is outweighed by the nutritional benefits.

When you have decided which plan is right for you, sit down for half an hour and write a shopping list, so you'll have everything you need for the first few days.

Make sure when you go shopping you take the 20:30:30:20 GDA values with you. These will help you make sure you're choosing the best cereals, ready meals, snacks and ingredients to help you reach your goals.

When you find the products which best fit the 20:30:30:20 guide, make a note of them for next time (see page 161). This will save you time in the coming weeks as you get more and more used to using the GDA labels to help you shop.

Money-saving tips

► Look out for special offers on fruit and vegetables – it's fine if you want to swap some of the fruit and veg in the plans to make the best use of bargains.
► Stock up on frozen vegetables too – they're just as nutritious as fresh, there's no waste and they will help you add more variety to your diet.

THE 7-DAY PLAN FOR BUSY PEOPLE
2000 Kcal plan

▶ All serving sizes are for 1 person.

▶ Ingredients are standard unless otherwise listed as low fat, reduced sugar, fat free etc.

▶ Ready-made meals or ingredients are indicated with an * asterisk.

> Please note that where the GDA for sugar exceeds 90 g for the day, any extra sugars are naturally occurring sugars and not added sugar. Many foods with naturally occurring sugars are excellent sources of vitamins, minerals and fibre and these nutritional benefits outweigh the slight excess in sugar. Any excess in natural sugars has been balanced by reductions in fat so that your total calories for the day remain within the GDA.

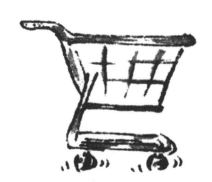

DAY 1
TOTAL GDA FOR THE DAY

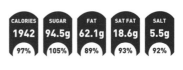

CALORIES	SUGAR	FAT	SAT FAT	SALT
1942	94.5g	62.1g	18.6g	5.5g
97%	105%	89%	93%	92%

Breakfast
150g melon
1 toasted English muffin, *and*
1 slice wholemeal toast *with*
3 tsp reduced fat spread *and*
2 tsp jam

CALORIES	SUGAR	FAT	SAT FAT	SALT
377	20.9g	9.7g	1.8g	1.0g
19%	23%	14%	9%	17%

Breakfast 20% GDA

First Snack
1 banana
1 tbsp low fat yogurt *with*
1 tbsp no added sugar muesli

CALORIES	SUGAR	FAT	SAT FAT	SALT
170	25.0g	1.6g	0.5g	0.1g
9%	28%	2%	3%	2%

Snack 10% GDA

Lunch
1 *Salmon and cucumber
    sandwich
Toasted tea cake *and*
1 tsp reduced fat spread
150 ml orange juice

CALORIES	SUGAR	FAT	SAT FAT	SALT
599	23.6g	17.4g	6.6g	2.1g
30%	26%	25%	33%	35%

Lunch 30% GDA

Second Snack
5 water biscuits *with*
3 tsp low fat soft cheese
Handful of grapes

CALORIES	SUGAR	FAT	SAT FAT	SALT
191	7.9g	7.0g	2.4g	0.5g
10%	9%	10%	12%	8%

Snack 10% GDA

Dinner
Vegetable crudités (choose 2 of
    the following: 1 carrot, 2
    sticks of celery, 1 red pepper,
    4 broccoli florets) *with*
1 tbsp *houmous
½ large, *ham and pineapple
    pizza *with*
a large dessert bowl of mixed
    salad *and*
1 tbsp *fat-free dressing

CALORIES	SUGAR	FAT	SAT FAT	SALT
605	17.1g	26.4g	7.3g	1.8g
30%	19%	38%	37%	30%

Dinner 30% GDA

DAY 2
TOTAL GDA FOR THE DAY

CALORIES	SUGAR	FAT	SAT FAT	SALT
1843	88.5g	48.3g	14.0g	6g
92%	98%	69%	70%	100%

Breakfast

½ grapefruit *with*
½ tsp sugar
50g corn flakes *with*
150ml semi-skimmed milk
1 slice wholegrain toast *with*
1 tsp reduced fat spread

CALORIES	SUGAR	FAT	SAT FAT	SALT
394	19.7g	7.2g	2.5g	1.2g
20%	22%	10%	13%	20%

Breakfast 20% GDA

First Snack

½ (15g) packet mini rice and corn snacks
1 small banana

CALORIES	SUGAR	FAT	SAT FAT	SALT
138	17.7g	1.4g	0.3g	0.5g
7%	20%	2%	2%	8%

Snack 10% GDA

Lunch

300g carton of *fresh Red Thai chicken soup *with*
2 small wholemeal rolls
2 Scotch pancakes *with*
80g strawberries

CALORIES	SUGAR	FAT	SAT FAT	SALT
547	26.4g	16.4g	3.3g	1.9g
27%	29%	23%	17%	32%

Lunch 30% GDA

Second Snack

4 water biscuits *with*
30g *low-fat pâté (any type)

CALORIES	SUGAR	FAT	SAT FAT	SALT
198	0.6g	12.5g	2.9g	0.7g
10%	0.7%	18%	15%	12%

Snack 10% GDA

Dinner

450g *potato-topped chicken and broccoli pie *with*
carrots and sweetcorn
80g stewed apple *with*
3 tbsp *low fat custard

CALORIES	SUGAR	FAT	SAT FAT	SALT
566	24.1g	10.8g	5.0g	1.7g
28%	27%	15%	25%	28%

Dinner 30% GDA

DAY 3
TOTAL GDA FOR THE DAY

CALORIES	SUGAR	FAT	SAT FAT	SALT
1981	95.1g	62.2g	17.9g	6g
99%	106%	89%	90%	100%

Breakfast
80g melon
60g no-added-sugar muesli *with*
2 rounded tbsp low fat natural
  yogurt
1 toasted crumpet *with*
1 tsp reduced fat spread

CALORIES	SUGAR	FAT	SAT FAT	SALT
396	21.0g	8.0g	1.7g	1.4g
20%	23%	11%	9%	23%

Breakfast 20% GDA

First Snack
1 mug *instant low-fat hot
  chocolate
1 Jaffa cake

CALORIES	SUGAR	FAT	SAT FAT	SALT
198	19.2g	7.3g	3.5g	0.3g
10%	21%	10%	18%	5%

Snack 10% GDA

Lunch
1 *egg and cress sandwich
1 banana
1 tbsp low fat yogurt *with*
1 tbsp no added sugar muesli

CALORIES	SUGAR	FAT	SAT FAT	SALT
581	26.7g	22.3g	5.5g	1.8g
29%	30%	32%	28%	30%

Lunch 30% GDA

Second Snack
Vegetable crudités (choose two
  of the following: 1 carrot, 2
  sticks of celery, 1 red pepper,
  4 broccoli florets)
2 bread sticks *with*
1 tbsp *houmous

CALORIES	SUGAR	FAT	SAT FAT	SALT
191	5.9g	12.1g	1.9g	0.9g
10%	7%	17%	10%	15%

Snack 10% GDA

Dinner
400g portion *spaghetti
  bolognese *with*
large dessert bowl of mixed
  salad *and*
1 tbsp *fat-free dressing
handful of fresh raspberries
2 tbsp oat granola *with*
1 tbsp low fat yogurt

CALORIES	SUGAR	FAT	SAT FAT	SALT
615	22.3g	12.5g	5.3g	1.6g
31%	25%	18%	27%	27%

Dinner 30% GDA

DAY 4
TOTAL GDA FOR THE DAY

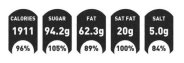

CALORIES	SUGAR	FAT	SAT FAT	SALT
1911	94.2g	62.3g	20g	5.0g
96%	105%	89%	100%	84%

Breakfast
35g ready-to-eat prunes
1 sachet instant porridge *with*
150ml semi skimmed milk
2 slices wholegrain toast *with*
2 tsp jam

CALORIES	SUGAR	FAT	SAT FAT	SALT
412	31.3g	6.9g	1.8g	0.7g
21%	35%	10%	9%	12%

Breakfast 20% GDA

First Snack
1 small (33g) *flapjack
1 slice fresh pineapple

CALORIES	SUGAR	FAT	SAT FAT	SALT
177	17.9g	6.3g	2.8g	0.01g
9%	20%	9%	14%	0.2%

Snack 10% GDA

Lunch
300g carton, *fresh tomato and
    basil soup *with* 1 granary bap
4 water biscuits *with* 30g brie
Small handful of grapes

CALORIES	SUGAR	FAT	SAT FAT	SALT
583	18.7g	19.3g	6.1g	2.5g
29%	21%	28%	31%	42%

Lunch 30% GDA

Second Snack
4 water biscuits *with*
2 tsp low fat soft cheese
80g melon

CALORIES	SUGAR	FAT	SAT FAT	SALT
138	3.7g	5.2g	1.3g	0.4g
7%	4%	7%	7%	7%

Snack 10% GDA

Dinner
100g *broccoli quiche *with*
200g boiled new potatoes *and*
2 × 80g servings of vegetables of
    choice *or*
large dessert bowl of mixed
    salad
2 *Scotch pancakes

CALORIES	SUGAR	FAT	SAT FAT	SALT
601	22.6g	24.6g	8.0g	1.4g
30%	25%	35%	40%	23%

Dinner 30% GDA

DAY 5
TOTAL GDA FOR THE DAY

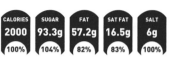

CALORIES	SUGAR	FAT	SAT FAT	SALT
2000	93.3g	57.2g	16.5g	6g
100%	104%	82%	83%	100%

Breakfast
60g puffed-wheat cereal *with*
150ml semi-skimmed milk
1 toasted crumpet *with* 1tsp
   reduce fat spread
Large handful of grapes

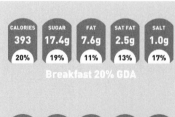

CALORIES	SUGAR	FAT	SAT FAT	SALT
393	17.4g	7.6g	2.5g	1.0g
20%	19%	11%	13%	17%

Breakfast 20% GDA

First Snack
1 toasted English muffin *and*
1tsp reduced fat spread

CALORIES	SUGAR	FAT	SAT FAT	SALT
201	3.1g	5.4g	1.1g	0.5g
10	3%	8%	6%	8%

Snack 10% GDA

Lunch
1 *tuna and sweetcorn sandwich
2tbsp oat granola *with*
1tbsp low fat yogurt *and*
handful of fresh raspberries

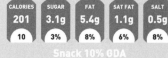

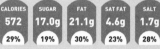

CALORIES	SUGAR	FAT	SAT FAT	SALT
572	17.0g	21.1g	4.6g	1.7g
29%	19%	30%	23%	28%

Lunch 30% GDA

Second Snack
2 Scotch pancakes *with*
1tbsp low-fat yogurt *and*
handful of blueberries

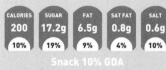

CALORIES	SUGAR	FAT	SAT FAT	SALT
200	17.2g	6.5g	0.8g	0.6g
10%	19%	9%	4%	10%

Snack 10% GDA

Dinner
450g *sausage and mash *with*
2 or 3 80g servings of vegetables
140g fruit salad *with*
1 scoop *soft-scoop vanilla ice
   cream

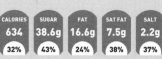

CALORIES	SUGAR	FAT	SAT FAT	SALT
634	38.6g	16.6g	7.5g	2.2g
32%	43%	24%	38%	37%

Dinner 30% GDA

DAY 6

TOTAL GDA FOR THE DAY

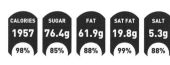

CALORIES	SUGAR	FAT	SAT FAT	SALT
1957	76.4g	61.9g	19.8g	5.3g
98%	85%	88%	99%	88%

Breakfast

125 ml fruit juice
30 g malted square cereal *with*
130 ml semi-skimmed milk
1 reduced fat croissant *with*
1 tsp marmalade

CALORIES	SUGAR	FAT	SAT FAT	SALT
389	29.7g	9.3g	5.2g	1.0g
19%	33%	13%	26%	17%

Breakfast 20% GDA

First Snack

8–10 grapes *and*
1 kiwi fruit
4 water biscuits *with*
1 tbsp cottage cheese

CALORIES	SUGAR	FAT	SAT FAT	SALT
172	12.0g	3.6g	0.4g	0.5g
9%	13%	5%	2%	8%

Snack 10% GDA

Lunch

1 *chicken caesar wrap
Banana

CALORIES	SUGAR	FAT	SAT FAT	SALT
595	25.5g	27.3g	4.7g	1.5g
30%	28%	39%	24%	25%

Lunch 30% GDA

Second Snack

2 slices wholemeal toast *with*
2 tsp reduced fat spread

CALORIES	SUGAR	FAT	SAT FAT	SALT
210	2.6g	8.1g	1.4g	0.7g
11%	3%	12%	7%	12%

Snack 10% GDA

Dinner

400 g*king prawn and vegetable
  masala *or*
*chicken curry *with (comes with
  rice)*
1 large (90 g) wholemeal pitta
  bread
1 satsuma

CALORIES	SUGAR	FAT	SAT FAT	SALT
591	6.6g	13.6g	8.1g	1.6g
30%	7%	19%	41%	27%

Dinner 30% GDA

DAY 7
TOTAL GDA FOR THE DAY

CALORIES	SUGAR	FAT	SAT FAT	SALT
1896	99.6g	54.2g	15.9g	3.2g
95%	111%	77%	80%	53%

Breakfast
30g prunes in fruit juice
2 × 27g sachets instant porridge *with*
300ml semi-skimmed milk

CALORIES	SUGAR	FAT	SAT FAT	SALT
359	19.7g	9.7g	4g	0.3g
18%	22%	14%	20%	5%

Breakfast 20% GDA

First Snack
1 sliced banana *with*
1 tbsp low-fat natural yogurt *and*
2 tbsp no-added-sugar muesli

CALORIES	SUGAR	FAT	SAT FAT	SALT
223	27.4g	2.5g	0.6g	0.2g
11%	30%	4%	3%	3%

Snack 10% GDA

Lunch
1 *individual chicken and pasta salad *with*
6–7 cherry tomatoes
5cm (2in) baguette
1 satsuma

CALORIES	SUGAR	FAT	SAT FAT	SALT
533	9.9g	16.9g	4.5g	1.3g
27%	11%	24%	23%	22%

Lunch 30% GDA

Second Snack
40g fruit cereal bar
80g melon

CALORIES	SUGAR	FAT	SAT FAT	SALT
161	20.7g	2.6g	1.0g	0.2g
8%	23%	4%	5%	3%

Snack 10% GDA

Dinner
3 slices roast beef with gravy (from oven-ready roasting joint)
4 tbsp mashed potato (fresh or ready-made)
2 × 80g servings of vegetables
60g *fruit crumble *and*
2 tbsp *reduced-fat custard

CALORIES	SUGAR	FAT	SAT FAT	SALT
620	21.9g	22.5g	5.8g	1.2g
31%	24%	32%	29%	20%

Dinner 30% GDA

THE 7-DAY PLAN FOR VEGETARIANS
2000 Kcal plan

▶ All serving sizes are a single portion for 1 person.

▶ Ingredients are standard unless otherwise listed as low fat, reduced sugar, fat free etc.

▶ Ready-made meals or ingredients are indicated by an * asterisk. Meals where recipes are provided are indicated in **bold**.

Please note that where the GDA for sugar exceeds 90g for the day, any extra sugars are naturally occurring sugars and not added sugar. Many foods with naturally occurring sugars are excellent sources of vitamins, minerals and fibre and these nutritional benefits outweigh the slight excess in sugar. Any excess in natural sugars has been balanced by reductions in fat so that your total calories for the day remain within the GDA.

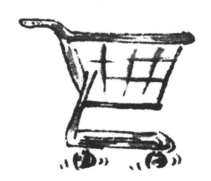

DAY 1
TOTAL GDA FOR THE DAY

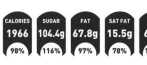

CALORIES	SUGAR	FAT	SAT FAT	SALT
1966	104.4g	67.8g	15.5g	6.0g
98%	116%	97%	78%	100%

Breakfast
½ grapefruit *with* 1 tsp sugar
1 low fat croissant
2 slices wholemeal toast *with*
1 tsp reduced fat spread *and* 2 tsp
   jam

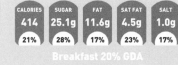

CALORIES	SUGAR	FAT	SAT FAT	SALT
414	25.1g	11.6g	4.5g	1.0g
21%	28%	17%	23%	17%

Breakfast 20% GDA

First Snack
250 ml *mango and strawberry
   smoothie

CALORIES	SUGAR	FAT	SAT FAT	SALT
158	20.9g	5.8g	3.7g	0.1g
8%	23%	8%	19%	2%

Snack 10% GDA

Lunch
300 g carton *mixed bean and
   tomato soup
1 large granary roll
1 toasted teacake *with*
1 tsp reduced-fat spread
handful of grapes

CALORIES	SUGAR	FAT	SAT FAT	SALT
575	28.0g	13.1g	2.8g	2.4g
29%	31%	19%	14%	40%

Lunch 30% GDA

Second Snack
Vegetable crudités (use 2 of the
   following: 1 carrot, 1 red
   pepper, 2 celery sticks, 4–5
   broccoli florets)
with 1 tbsp *houmous
½ toasted pitta bread, cut into
   strips

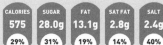

CALORIES	SUGAR	FAT	SAT FAT	SALT
223	6.4g	11.7g	1.4g	1.0g
11%	7%	17%	7%	17%

Snack 10% GDA

Dinner
1 nutty chickpea burger *with*
1 pitta bread
a large dessert bowl of mixed
   salad *with*
2 tsp *fat-free dressing
1 banana

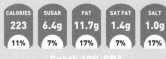

CALORIES	SUGAR	FAT	SAT FAT	SALT
596	24.0g	25.6g	3.1g	1.5g
30%	27%	37%	16%	25%

Dinner 30% GDA

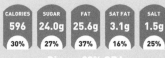

DAY 1 RECIPE

Nutty chickpea burgers (makes 10)

2 × 400 g cans chick peas in
   unsalted water
2 tbsp sesame oil
2 tbsp tahini
Large bunch fresh mint,
   chopped
4 tbsp mixed walnuts, almonds,
   sunflower seeds, mixed and
   crushed
flour for dusting
1 egg, beaten

1 Drain the chick peas and put in a food processor together with the sesame oil, tahini and fresh mint.

2 Blend to a smooth paste and form into approximately 10 patties.

3 Dust each patty with flour and dip in beaten egg. Coat with the crushed walnuts, almonds and sunflower seeds.

4 Refrigerate for an hour.

5 Grill under a medium heat, or dry fry gently in a non-stick pan for 5 minutes until golden.

Can be frozen.

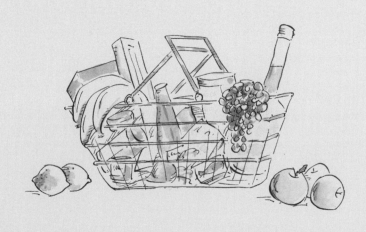

DAY 2
TOTAL GDA FOR THE DAY

CALORIES	SUGAR	FAT	SAT FAT	SALT
1971	92.3g	61.6g	17.2g	6.0g
99%	103%	88%	86%	100%

Breakfast
50 g puffed wheat cereal *with*
150 ml semi-skimmed milk *and*
2 tbsp blueberries
1 toasted crumpet *with* 1 tsp
reduced fat spread

CALORIES	SUGAR	FAT	SAT FAT	SALT
405	16g	7.7g	2.5g	1.1g
20%	18%	7%	10%	18%

Breakfast 20% GDA

First Snack
1 tbsp *guacamole
3 rye crispbreads
1 apple

CALORIES	SUGAR	FAT	SAT FAT	SALT
193	12.6g	5.7g	1.2g	0.3g
10%	14%	8%	6%	5%

Snack 10% GDA

Lunch
1 *egg and salad sandwich on
    wholemeal bread
1 bag mini rye crispbread snacks
1 [40 g] dried fruit and cereal bar
1 peach or nectarine

CALORIES	SUGAR	FAT	SAT FAT	SALT
605	33.6g	18.4g	4.9g	1.7g
30%	37%	26%	25%	28%

Lunch 30% GDA

Second Snack
1 slice wholemeal toast *with*
1 tsp jam *and*
1 heaped tsp peanut butter

CALORIES	SUGAR	FAT	SAT FAT	SALT
195	7.5g	9.2g	2.2g	0.4g
10%	8%	13%	11%	7%

Snack 10% GDA

Dinner
350 g *vegetable lasagne
a large mixed salad *and*
1 tbsp *Caesar dressing *and*
10 g parmesan shavings *with*
5 cm (2 in) chunk of baguette
1 satsuma

CALORIES	SUGAR	FAT	SAT FAT	SALT
573	22.6g	20.6g	6.4g	2.5g
29%	25%	29%	32%	42%

Dinner 30% GDA

DAY 3
TOTAL GDA FOR THE DAY

CALORIES	SUGAR	FAT	SAT FAT	SALT
1982	92.2g	70.0g	20g	5.9g
99%	102%	100%	100%	98%

Breakfast
3 wheat biscuits *with*
170 ml semi-skimmed milk
1 slice wholegrain toast *with*
1 tsp honey
handful of sliced strawberries

CALORIES	SUGAR	FAT	SAT FAT	SALT
411	22.0g	5.1g	2.3g	0.8g
21%	24%	7%	12%	13%

Breakfast 20% GDA

First Snack
Avocado and tomato salad
2 bread sticks

CALORIES	SUGAR	FAT	SAT FAT	SALT
212	4.7g	15.4g	4.2g	0.3g
11%	5%	22%	21%	5%

Snack 10% GDA

Lunch
1 wholemeal pitta bread *filled with*
3 *mini falafel bites
Greek salad *and*
1 tsp *fat-free dressing
1 sliced banana *with*
2 tbsp low-fat yogurt *and*
1 tbsp granola

CALORIES	SUGAR	FAT	SAT FAT	SALT
575	36.4g	17.7g	6.0g	3.1g
29%	40%	25%	30%	52%

Lunch 30% GDA

Second Snack
1 slice wholegrain toast *with*
1 tsp jam *and* 1 heaped tsp
   peanut butter

CALORIES	SUGAR	FAT	SAT FAT	SALT
195	7.5g	9.2g	2.2g	0.4g
10%	8%	13%	11%	7%

Snack 10% GDA

Dinner
120 g *broccoli, tomato and
   cheese quiche *with*
200 g boiled new potatoes *and*
2 × 100 g vegetables of choice *or*
a large dessert bowl of mixed
   salad
2 *Scotch pancakes

CALORIES	SUGAR	FAT	SAT FAT	SALT
589	21.6g	22.6g	5.3g	1.3g
29%	24%	32%	27%	22%

Dinner 30% GDA

DAY 3 RECIPES

Greek salad

120 g iceberg lettuce
2 tomatoes
¼ cucumber
50 g feta cheese
4–5 black olives

1 Shred the lettuce into thin strips.

2 Dice the tomatoes and the cucumber

3 Cube the feta cheese into bite-sized chunks

4 Slice the olives

5 Mix all ingredients lightly in a bowl and serve.

Avocado and tomato salad

½ ripe avocado
2 tomatoes
1 tsp olive oil
1 tbsp balsamic vinegar
a squeeze of lemon juice

1 Peel the avocado, remove the stone, and dice into bit-sized pieces.

2 Roughly dice the tomatoes.

3 Mix the avocado and the tomatoes gently in a bowl.

4 Add the olive oil, balsamic vinegar and lemon juice.

5 To eat at its best, serve as soon as possible.

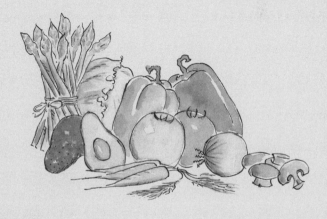

DAY 4
TOTAL GDA FOR THE DAY

CALORIES	SUGAR	FAT	SAT FAT	SALT
2000	92.7g	47.0g	15.6g	4.4g
100%	103%	67%	78%	73%

Breakfast
50g corn flakes *with*
150ml semi-skimmed milk
1 slice wholegrain toast *with*
1 tsp reduced-fat spread
½ grapefruit with 1 tsp sugar

CALORIES	SUGAR	FAT	SAT FAT	SALT
401	21.7g	7.2g	2.5g	1.2g
20%	24%	10%	13%	20%

Breakfast 20% GDA

First Snack
80g melon
1 toasted English muffin *with*
1 tsp reduced fat spread

CALORIES	SUGAR	FAT	SAT FAT	SALT
216	6.3g	5.5g	1.1g	0.6g
11%	7%	8%	6%	10%

Snack 10% GDA

Lunch
1 large baked potato *with* 2 tsp
   reduced-fat spread *and*
1 small tin baked beans (reduced
   sugar and salt variety), heated
1 tbsp low fat yogurt *with*
1 tbsp no added sugar muesli *and*
1 sliced banana

CALORIES	SUGAR	FAT	SAT FAT	SALT
585	36.4g	8.9g	1.7g	1.4g
29%	40%	13%	9%	23%

Lunch 30% GDA

Second Snack
4 water biscuits *with* 40g
   *mushroom pâté
1 apple

CALORIES	SUGAR	FAT	SAT FAT	SALT
206	12.1g	8.4g	2.0g	0.3g
10%	13%	12%	10%	5%

Snack 10% GDA

Dinner
**Broad bean, beetroot and goats
   cheese salad** *with*
80g (dry weight) brown rice,
   cooked
1 kiwi fruit

CALORIES	SUGAR	FAT	SAT FAT	SALT
592	16.2g	17.0g	8.3g	0.9g
30%	18%	24%	42%	15%

Dinner 30% GDA

DAY 4 RECIPE

Broad bean, beetroot and goats cheese salad

2 tbsp broad beans, podded or frozen
½ shallot, diced
1 clove garlic, finely sliced
1 tbsp olive oil
2 medium sized beetroot, cooked and quartered
½ tsp fresh rosemary, chopped
1 tbsp red wine vinegar
A large dessert bowl of mixed salad leaves
40 g goats cheese, sliced

1 Boil the broad beans until cooked, and refresh in cold water.

2 Lightly fry the shallot and the garlic in the olive oil until lightly browned.

3 Add the beetroot and rosemary and warm over a gentle heat for 3–4 minutes.

4 Stir in 1 tbsp red wine vinegar and pour the beetroot mixture over the bowl of mixed salad leaves.

5 Top with the broad beans and goats cheese.

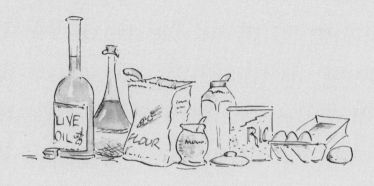

DAY 5
TOTAL GDA FOR THE DAY

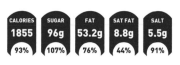

CALORIES	SUGAR	FAT	SAT FAT	SALT
1855	96g	53.2g	8.8g	5.5g
93%	107%	76%	44%	91%

Breakfast
80g pineapple
60g no-added-sugar muesli
2 tbsp low-fat natural yogurt
1 slice wholemeal toast *with*
1 tsp reduced-fat spread

CALORIES	SUGAR	FAT	SAT FAT	SALT
402	23.4g	9.7g	2.1g	0.5g
20%	26%	14%	11%	8%

Breakfast 20% GDA

First Snack
3 rye crispbreads
1½ tbsp cottage cheese
Small bunch grapes

CALORIES	SUGAR	FAT	SAT FAT	SALT
183	10.0g	2.6g	1.4g	0.6g
9%	11%	4%	7%	10%

Snack 10% GDA

Lunch
Roasted vegetable and houmous wrap
1 tbsp natural yogurt *with*
2 tbsp rolled oats *and*
1 small banana

CALORIES	SUGAR	FAT	SAT FAT	SALT
600	29.5g	18.1g	2.8g	1.5g
30%	33%	26%	14%	25%

Lunch 30% GDA

Second Snack
12 almonds *and*
1 peach or nectarine

CALORIES	SUGAR	FAT	SAT FAT	SALT
186	8.2g	14g	1.1g	0.06g
9%	9%	20%	6%	1%

Snack 10% GDA

Dinner
Spaghetti bolognese with Quorn™ mince
with a large mixed salad *and*
1 tbsp *fat-free dressing
1 large orange

CALORIES	SUGAR	FAT	SAT FAT	SALT
484	24.9g	8.8g	1.4g	2.8g
24%	28%	13%	7%	47%

Dinner 30% GDA

DAY 5 RECIPES

Roasted vegetable wrap

1 *tortilla wrap
1 tbsp *houmous
200 g vegetables of choice:
   peppers, onions, aubergines,
   sweet potatoes, mushrooms,
   washed and diced
1 tbsp olive oil
1 tsp *Cajun seasoning

1 Chop the vegetables into
2.5 cm (1 in) chunks.

2 Toss, in the oil and Cajun
seasoning.

3 Roast in a hot oven (Gas mark
6, 200 °C) for 20–25 minutes.

4 Spread the houmous over one
side of the wrap.

5 Add the hot roasted
vegetables.

6 Roll up the wrap, taking care
to fold in one end to prevent the
filling from falling out.

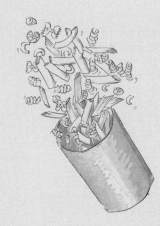

Spaghetti bolognese with Quorn™ mince

¼ onion, diced
a little olive oil
87 g Quorn mince
200 g jar *bolognese sauce
100 g (dry weight) pasta

1 Gently soften the onion in a little
olive oil. Add Quorn mince and heat
through.

2 Pour in bolognese sauce and
heat gently until bubbling. Stir
occasionally.

3 Cook pasta according to packet
instructions.

4 Drain pasta and serve,
smothered in the bolognese sauce.

DAY 6
TOTAL GDA FOR THE DAY

CALORIES	SUGAR	FAT	SAT FAT	SALT
1890	73.9g	67.0g	19.4g	5.3g
95%	82%	96%	97%	88%

Breakfast
125 ml fruit juice
1½ eggs scrambled *with*
2 tbsp semi-skimmed milk
2 slices wholegrain toast *with*
2 grilled tomatoes *and*
2 tbsp grilled sliced mushrooms

CALORIES	SUGAR	FAT	SAT FAT	SALT
405	18.5g	14.9g	4.3g	0.8g
20%	21%	21%	22%	13%

Breakfast 20% GDA

First Snack
2 tbsp *tzatziki *with*
vegetable crudités (choose 2
    from: 1 carrot, 1 yellow
    pepper, 4 broccoli florets,
    2 celery sticks)
4 bread sticks
1 orange

CALORIES	SUGAR	FAT	SAT FAT	SALT
198	17.2g	5.1g	1.2g	0.7g
10%	19%	7%	6%	12%

Snack 10% GDA

Lunch
Vegetarian niçoise salad *with*
5 cm (2 in) baguette
1 toasted tea cake *and*
2 tsp reduced-fat spread

CALORIES	SUGAR	FAT	SAT FAT	SALT
590	16.0g	24.8g	6.7g	1.8g
30%	18%	35%	34%	30%

Lunch 30% GDA

Second Snack
2 Dutch crispbakes *topped with*
Lentil and tomato salad

CALORIES	SUGAR	FAT	SAT FAT	SALT
219	5.2g	6.9g	1.1g	0.9g
11%	6%	10%	6%	15%

Snack 10% GDA

Dinner
½ *margarita pizza (410 g) *with*
a large dessert bowl of mixed
    salad *and*
1 tbsp *fat-free dressing
1 satsuma

CALORIES	SUGAR	FAT	SAT FAT	SALT
478	17.0g	15.3g	6.1g	1.1g
24%	19%	22%	31%	18%

Dinner 30% GDA

DAY 6 RECIPES

Lentil and tomato salad

80g tin of lentils, rinsed and
    drained
¼ red pepper, finely diced
3 cherry tomatoes
1 spring onion, sliced
15g olives, black or green
1 tsp olive oil
1 tsp balsamic vinegar

1 Combine the lentils with all the salad ingredients.

2 Drizzle over the olive oil and balsamic vinegar. Stir well.

Vegetarian niçoise salad

150g new potatoes
¼ iceberg lettuce
50g green beans
5 cherry tomatoes
2 spring onions, sliced
15g black olives
2 eggs, hard-boiled, peeled and
    quartered
50g smoked or plain tofu, diced

1 Boil the new potatoes and green beans, and quarter them.

2 Shred a generous serving of iceberg lettuce.

3 Mix potatoes, beans and lettuce together with the tomatoes and spring onions.

4 Add the olives and hard-boiled eggs, and top with the tofu.

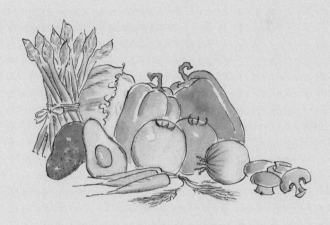

DAY 7
TOTAL GDA FOR THE DAY

CALORIES	SUGAR	FAT	SAT FAT	SALT
1874	104.5g	70g	16.3g	6g
94%	116%	100%	83%	100%

Breakfast
Porridge *made with*
60g oats *and*
250ml semi-skimmed milk
topped with
1 tbsp raisins tossed in cinnamon

CALORIES	SUGAR	FAT	SAT FAT	SALT
377	21.7g	9.6g	3.8g	0.2g
19%	24%	14%	19%	3%

Breakfast 20% GDA

First Snack
2 Scotch pancakes
1 apple

CALORIES	SUGAR	FAT	SAT FAT	SALT
214	23.0g	6.1g	0.5g	0.4g
11%	26%	9%	3%	7%

Snack 10% GDA

Lunch
**Spinach, feta cheese and
     mushroom omelette** *with*
a large mixed salad *and*
1 tbsp **low-fat vinaigrette** *and*
1 large wholemeal roll
1 banana

CALORIES	SUGAR	FAT	SAT FAT	SALT
552	25.5g	26.1g	9.4g	2.8g
28%	28%	37%	47%	47%

Lunch 30% GDA

Second Snack
9 almonds *and* 1 orange

CALORIES	SUGAR	FAT	SAT FAT	SALT
175	13.7g	10.7g	0.98g	0.02g
9%	15%	15%	4%	0%

Snack 10% GDA

Dinner
**Falafel and lemon couscous with
     a tomato salad**
140g mixed berries *with*
2 tbsp low fat yogurt

CALORIES	SUGAR	FAT	SAT FAT	SALT
556	20.6g	17.5g	2.1g	2.6g
28%	23%	25%	11%	43%

Dinner 30% GDA

DAY 7 RECIPES

Low-fat vinaigrette

See page 169

Spinach, feta cheese and mushroom omelette

1 tsp sunflower oil
75 g mushrooms, sliced
2 handfuls baby spinach leaves, washed
40 g feta cheese, cut into small chunks
2 eggs, beaten
20 ml milk
ground black pepper to season

1 Warm the oil over a low heat in a non-stick frying pan.

2 Fry the mushrooms for 3–4 minutes, until soft.

3 Combine all the other ingredients and add to the pan with the mushrooms.

4 Heat gently until golden brown underneath.

Serve immediately.

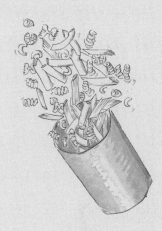

Falafel and lemon couscous with a tomato salad

2 tomatoes, chopped into chunks
1 tsp olive oil
½ tsp ground paprika
½ tsp ground cumin
handful of mint, chopped
180 g *couscous, lemon flavoured
4 *falafel

1 Combine tomatoes, olive oil, paprika, cumin and mint. Stir well.

2 Prepare couscous according to the packet instructions.

3 Warm falafel in a hot oven (Gas mark 6, 200 °C) for 10–15 minutes.

4 Top the couscous with the falafel and serve the tomato salad on the side.

► All serving sizes are for 1 person.

► Ingredients are standard unless otherwise listed as low fat, reduced sugar, fat free etc.

► Ready-made meals or ingredients are indicated with an * asterisk. Meals where recipes are provided are indicated in **bold**. *See the at glance 7 day plan table for all the budget ranges used, shown in italics.*

Please note that where the GDA for sugar exceeds 90 g for the day, any extra sugars are naturally occurring sugars and not added sugar. Many foods with naturally occurring sugars are excellent sources of vitamins, minerals and fibre and these nutritional benefits outweigh the slight excess in sugar. Any excess in natural sugars has been balanced by reductions in fat so that your total calories for the day remain within the GDA.

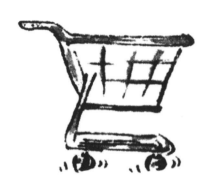

Diet tips for cooking on a budget

► Jam, marmalade and honey can be used interchangeably.

► Buy seasonal fruits and vegetables to keep costs down and stock up with frozen fruit and vegetables. Frozen fruit and veg is just as nutritious as fresh and means you don't have so much waste.

► Look out for bulk buys on foods you usually purchase that fit in with the GDA profile.

► Cook from scratch more often – ready meals are more expensive than preparing your own because you are paying someone else to do the work.

► Make bulk batches of meals when you buy foods on offer and freeze in family-sized or individual portions.

Average portion sizes are included in savvy GDA tips (see page 177).

DAY 1
TOTAL GDA FOR THE DAY

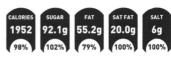

CALORIES	SUGAR	FAT	SAT FAT	SALT
1952	92.1g	55.2g	20.0g	6g
98%	102%	79%	100%	100%

Breakfast
100g canned grapefruit segments
   in light syrup
45g cornflakes *with*
150ml semi-skimmed milk
1 slice wholemeal toast *with*
1 tsp reduced fat spread

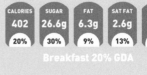

CALORIES	SUGAR	FAT	SAT FAT	SALT
402	26.6g	6.3g	2.6g	1.3g
20%	30%	9%	13%	22%

Breakfast 20% GDA

First Snack
1 apple
handful of grapes
3 tbsp natural yogurt

CALORIES	SUGAR	FAT	SAT FAT	SALT
166	26.0g	3.7g	2.0g	0.2g
8%	29%	5%	10%	3%

Snack 10% GDA

Lunch
140g can *mixed tuna and
   sweetcorn *with*
1 tbsp *reduced-fat salad cream
   and
2 slices wholemeal bread
1 sultana scone *with* 1 tsp
   reduced-fat spread *and* 1 tsp
   jam

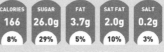

CALORIES	SUGAR	FAT	SAT FAT	SALT
582	19.4g	14.6g	3.9g	2.4g
29%	22%	21%	20%	40%

Lunch 30% GDA

Second Snack
3 rye crackers *with*
30g *low-fat pâté

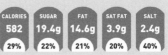

CALORIES	SUGAR	FAT	SAT FAT	SALT
197	1.0g	7.6g	2.5g	0.7g
10%	1%	11%	13%	12%

Snack 10% GDA

Dinner
100g *cheese and bacon quiche
   with
240g (8) new potatoes *and*
a large dessert bowl of mixed
   salad *or*
2 × 80g servings of vegetables
140g stewed fruit *with*
2 tbsp *custard
1 digestive biscuit

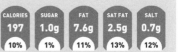

CALORIES	SUGAR	FAT	SAT FAT	SALT
605	19.1g	23.0g	9.0g	1.4g
30%	21%	33%	45%	16%

Dinner 30% GDA

DAY 2
TOTAL GDA FOR THE DAY

CALORIES 1998 100%

SUGAR 98.1g 109%

FAT 54.6g 78%

SAT FAT 20g 100%

SALT 4.3g 71%

Breakfast
3 tbsp muesli with
140 ml semi-skimmed milk
125 ml breakfast juice
1 slice wholemeal toast *with*
1 tsp reduced fat spread

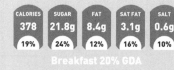

CALORIES 378 19% | **SUGAR** 21.8g 24% | **FAT** 8.4g 12% | **SAT FAT** 3.1g 16% | **SALT** 0.6g 10%

Breakfast 20% GDA

First Snack
1 muesli cereal bar
2 small satsumas
1 rich tea biscuit

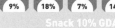

CALORIES 187 9% | **SUGAR** 16.2g 18% | **FAT** 5.2g 7% | **SAT FAT** 2.7g 14% | **SALT** 0.3g 5%

Snack 10% GDA

Lunch
1 large baked potato *with*
200 g baked beans heated *and*
25 g grated cheese
1 *Scotch pancake

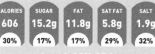

CALORIES 606 30% | **SUGAR** 15.2g 17% | **FAT** 11.8g 17% | **SAT FAT** 5.8g 29% | **SALT** 1.9g 32%

Lunch 30% GDA

Second Snack
2 tbsp natural yogurt *and*
2 tbsp oats *with*
1 large banana, sliced

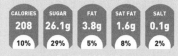

CALORIES 208 10% | **SUGAR** 26.1g 29% | **FAT** 3.8g 5% | **SAT FAT** 1.6g 8% | **SALT** 0.1g 2%

Snack 10% GDA

Dinner
1 medium pork chop, grilled
1 tsp *apple sauce
3 scoops mashed potato *and*
2 × 80 g servings of vegetables
    with
gravy
25 g milk chocolate

CALORIES 619 31% | **SUGAR** 18.8g 21% | **FAT** 25.4g 36% | **SAT FAT** 6.8g 34% | **SALT** 1.4g 23%

Dinner 30% GDA

2000 kcal plan ON A BUDGET

DAY 3
TOTAL GDA FOR THE DAY

 CALORIES **1883** 94%
 SUGAR **97.4g** 108%
 FAT **49.7g** 71%
 SAT FAT **13.8g** 69%
 SALT **6g** 100%

Breakfast

30g rice krispies *with*
140ml semi-skimmed milk
½ grapefruit *with* 1tsp sugar
2 slices wholemeal toast *with*
2tsp reduced-fat spread *and*
1tsp yeast extract

 CALORIES **426** 21%
 SUGAR **20.3g** 23%
 FAT **9.9g** 14%
 SAT FAT **3.9g** 20%
 SALT **1.0g** 17%

Breakfast 20% GDA

First Snack

1 sultana scone *with*
1tsp reduced-fat spread *and*
1tsp jam

 CALORIES **177** 9%
 SUGAR **9.4g** 10%
 FAT **6.4g** 9%
 SAT FAT **2.1g** 11%
SALT **0.5g** 8%

Snack 10% GDA

Lunch

200g can tomato soup *with*
2 small bread rolls
1 teacake *with*
1tsp reduced fat spread
1 apple

 CALORIES **534** 27%
 SUGAR **30.8g** 34%
 FAT **11.4g** 16%
SAT FAT **2.8g** 14%
SALT **2.7g** 45%

Lunch 30% GDA

Second Snack

5 bread sticks *with*
1tbsp cottage cheese
Vegetable crudités (choose 2
    from 1 carrot, 1 yellow
    pepper, 4 broccoli florets,
    2 celery sticks)

 CALORIES **145** 7%
 SUGAR **7.3g** 8%
 FAT **3.9g** 6%
 SAT FAT **2.5g** 13%
SALT **0.9g** 15%

Snack 10% GDA

Dinner
Chicken and vegetable stir fry
140g fruit salad

 CALORIES **601** 30%
 SUGAR **29.6g** 33%
 FAT **18.1g** 26%
 SAT FAT **2.5g** 13%
SALT **0.9g** 15%

Dinner 30% GDA

DAY 3 RECIPE

Chicken and vegetable stir fry

1 chicken breast boneless, skinless
1 tbsp water
selection of dried spices (e.g. chilli, all spice, Chinese 5 spice)
300 g mixed vegetables (raw) choose from: mangetout, baby corn, bean sprouts, thinly sliced peppers, sliced mushrooms
1 tsp sesame oil
1 tsp soy sauce
A sprinkling of sesame seeds
250 g noodles

1 Cut the chicken into 2.5 cm (1 in) pieces and sprinkle with the dried spices.

2 In a large frying pan or wok, heat 1 tbsp water, add the chicken pieces and toss around the pan until all of the chicken is sealed.

3 Add the prepared vegetables and continue to stir for 6–7 minutes.

4 Meanwhile heat a pan of water to cook the noodles according to the pack instructions. Usually 5–6 minutes.

5 Mix the sesame oil, soy sauce and sesame seeds.

6 Add the sesame mixture to the chicken and vegetables and when the liquid is piping hot serve over the drained, cooked noodles.

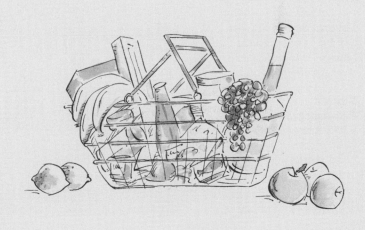

DAY 4
TOTAL GDA FOR THE DAY

CALORIES	SUGAR	FAT	SAT FAT	SALT
1906	98.8g	64.2g	20g	6g
95%	110%	92%	100%	100%

Breakfast
50g prunes in fruit juice
2 × 27g sachets of instant
   porridge *with*
300ml semi-skimmed milk

CALORIES	SUGAR	FAT	SAT FAT	SALT
375	23.5g	9.7g	4.0g	0.3g
19%	26%	14%	20%	5%

Breakfast 20% GDA

First Snack
Vegetable crudités (choose two
   from: 1 carrot, 1 yellow
   pepper, 4 broccoli florets,
   2 celery sticks) *with*
1 tbsp *houmous *and*
4 water biscuits

CALORIES	SUGAR	FAT	SAT FAT	SALT
245	7.1g	12.9g	2.0g	0.9g
12%	8%	18%	10%	15%

Snack 10% GDA

Lunch
1 *roast beef and horseradish
   sandwich on wholemeal bread
small salad of rocket leaves *and*
1 sliced tomato
1 × 125g pot fruit yogurt
1 toasted crumpet *with*
1 tsp reduced fat spread

CALORIES	SUGAR	FAT	SAT FAT	SALT
525	26.8g	12.5g	5.4g	1.8g
26%	30%	18%	27%	30%

Lunch 30% GDA

Second Snack
2 digestive biscuits *with*
1 mug of *low-calorie instant hot
   chocolate

CALORIES	SUGAR	FAT	SAT FAT	SALT
199	30.7g	5.4g	3.8g	0.1g
10%	34%	8%	19%	2%

Snack 10% GDA

Dinner
Pasta bolognese *with*
a large dessert bowl of mixed
   salad *and*
1 tbsp *fat-free dressing

CALORIES	SUGAR	FAT	SAT FAT	SALT
562	10.7g	23.7g	4.8g	2.9g
28%	12%	34%	24%	48%

Dinner 30% GDA

DAY 4 RECIPE

Pasta bolognese

110g turkey or pork mince, raw
½ onion, diced
handful of mushrooms, sliced
150g *bolognese sauce
80g (dry weight) spaghetti or
pasta shapes

1 Dry fry the mince in a non-stick pan, stirring all the time until it begins to brown.

2 Add the onion and mushrooms and continue to stir, cook for 6–7 minutes until softened.

3 Add bolognese sauce and simmer gently for 10 minutes.

4 Cook the pasta according to packet instructions.

Serve cooked bolognese on a bed of pasta.

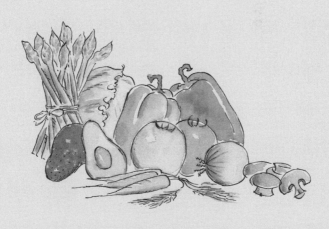

DAY 5
TOTAL GDA FOR THE DAY

CALORIES	SUGAR	FAT	SAT FAT	SALT
1928	102.8g	50.7g	16.7g	5.7g
96%	114%	72%	84%	95%

Breakfast
125 ml orange juice
1 English muffin toasted *with*
2 tsp reduced-fat spread
2 tbsp low fat plain yoghurt with
    80 g (defrosted) frozen mixed
    berries

CALORIES	SUGAR	FAT	SAT FAT	SALT
346	21.4g	8.0g	2.8g	0.8g
17%	24%	11%	14%	13%

Breakfast 20% GDA

First Snack
large handful of grapes
4 rye crispbread topped *with*
40 g reduced fat cream or soft
    cheese

CALORIES	SUGAR	FAT	SAT FAT	SALT
219	12.1g	3.9g	2.2g	0.6g
11%	13%	6%	11%	10%

Snack 10% GDA

Lunch
Egg and new potato salad
1 *Scotch pancake

CALORIES	SUGAR	FAT	SAT FAT	SALT
565	19.0g	21.3g	4.6g	1.1g
28%	21%	30%	23%	18%

Lunch 30% GDA

Second Snack
40 g bran flakes *with*
140 ml semi-skimmed milk *and*
6 sliced strawberries

CALORIES	SUGAR	FAT	SAT FAT	SALT
211	17.2g	3.3g	1.6g	0.7g
11%	19%	5%	8%	12%

Snack 10% GDA

Dinner
1 individual *margarita pizza (or
    190 g slice from a large
    margarita pizza) *with*
80 g vegetables as extra toppings
    (e.g. sliced peppers, onion,
    mushrooms) *and*
a large dessert bowl of green
    salad *and*
1 tbsp *fat-free dressing
1 banana

CALORIES	SUGAR	FAT	SAT FAT	SALT
587	33.1g	14.2g	5.5g	2.5g
29%	37%	20%	28%	42%

Dinner 30% GDA

DAY 5 RECIPE

Egg and new potato salad

2 eggs
6 new potatoes
2 tbsp reduced-fat salad cream
a large dessert bowl of mixed
   salad

1 Bring the eggs and potatoes to
the boil in separate pans.

2 Allow the new potatoes to
simmer for 20 minutes until
cooked. Drain and dice into
cubes.

3 Remove the eggs from the heat
and stand for 15 minutes.

4 Drain hot water and allow to
stand in cold water until completely
cooled before removing shells.

5 Slice the eggs, and mix together
with the eggs, potatoes and salad
cream.

Serve on a bed of salad.

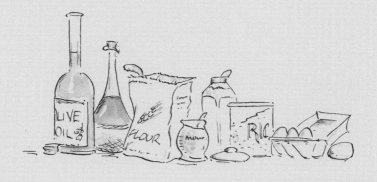

DAY 6
TOTAL GDA FOR THE DAY

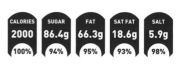

CALORIES	SUGAR	FAT	SAT FAT	SALT
2000	86.4g	66.3g	18.6g	5.9g
100%	94%	95%	93%	98%

Breakfast

1 toasted English muffin *with*
2 eggs, scrambled gently, in non-stick pan, with no added butter or milk *and*
2 tbsp baked beans (reduced sugar and salt), heated
125 ml orange juice

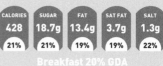

CALORIES	SUGAR	FAT	SAT FAT	SALT
428	18.7g	13.4g	3.7g	1.3g
21%	21%	19%	19%	22%

Breakfast 20% GDA

First Snack

2 tbsp natural yogurt and 3 tbsp oats *with*
1 small banana, sliced

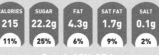

CALORIES	SUGAR	FAT	SAT FAT	SALT
215	22.2g	4.3g	1.7g	0.1g
11%	25%	6%	9%	2%

Snack 10% GDA

Lunch

2 *vegetarian burgers *with*
170 g **roasted potato wedges** *with*
1 tbsp *tomato salsa *or* chutney *and*
1 corn on the cob *and*
1 tsp low-fat spread

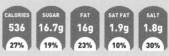

CALORIES	SUGAR	FAT	SAT FAT	SALT
536	16.7g	16g	1.9g	1.8g
27%	19%	23%	10%	30%

Lunch 30% GDA

Second Snack

30 g mixed unsalted nuts
1 tbsp raisins

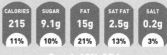

CALORIES	SUGAR	FAT	SAT FAT	SALT
215	9.1g	15g	2.5g	0.2g
11%	10%	21%	13%	3%

Snack 10% GDA

Dinner

300 g *beef lasagne with
a large bowl of mixed salad *and*
1 tbsp fat free dressing *and*
5 cm (2 in) baguette
handful of grapes
23 g oat and fruit cereal bar

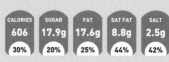

CALORIES	SUGAR	FAT	SAT FAT	SALT
606	17.9g	17.6g	8.8g	2.5g
30%	20%	25%	44%	42%

Dinner 30% GDA

DAY 6 RECIPE

Roasted potato wedges

170 g potatoes, unpeeled
Spray oil
1 tsp Cajun seasoning

1 Cut the potatoes into thick wedges – approx 1 cm (½ in). Keep their skins on.

2 Place wedges in a baking tray, sprinkle with Cajun seasoning and spray with oil.

3 Toss until the wedges are evenly coated.

4 Cook in a hot oven (Gas mark 6, 200 °C) for 30–35 minutes until lightly browned.

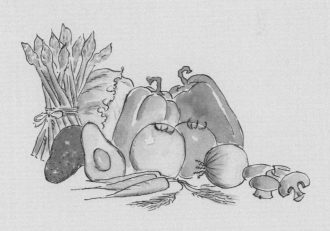

DAY 7
TOTAL GDA FOR THE DAY

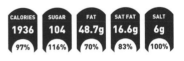

CALORIES	SUGAR	FAT	SAT FAT	SALT
1936	104	48.7g	16.6g	6g
97%	116%	70%	83%	100%

Breakfast
40 g puffed wheat cereal *with*
140 ml semi-skimmed milk
1 low-fat croissant *with* 1 tsp jam
80 g grapefruit segments in light
   syrup

CALORIES	SUGAR	FAT	SAT FAT	SALT
437	28.5g	10.1g	5.4g	0.6g
22%	32%	14%	27%	10%

Breakfast 20% GDA

First Snack
2 slices wholemeal toast *with*
2 tsp reduced-fat spread *and*
a scraping of yeast extract

CALORIES	SUGAR	FAT	SAT FAT	SALT
207	2.8g	6.4g	2.2g	1.2g
10%	3%	9%	11%	20%

Snack 10% GDA

Lunch
6 tbsp baked beans, heated *with*
2 slices wholemeal toast *with*
2 tsp reduced-fat spread
1 tbsp natural yogurt and 3 tbsp
   oats *with*
1 small banana, sliced

CALORIES	SUGAR	FAT	SAT FAT	SALT
547	32.2g	10.9g	3.4g	2g
27%	36%	16%	17%	33%

Lunch 30% GDA

Second Snack
2 *Scotch pancakes *with*
60 g mandarin segments in light
   syrup

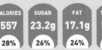

CALORIES	SUGAR	FAT	SAT FAT	SALT
188	17.3g	4.2g	0.4g	0.7g
9%	19%	6%	2%	12%

Snack 10% GDA

Dinner
Beef casserole *with*
3 scoops mashed potato (fresh or
   instant) *and*
3 × 80 g portions steamed
   vegetables
23 g muesli bar
1 apple

CALORIES	SUGAR	FAT	SAT FAT	SALT
557	23.2g	17.1g	5.2g	1.5g
28%	26%	24%	26%	25%

Dinner 30% GDA

DAY 7 RECIPE

Beef casserole

90 g lean stewing steak, cubed
½ onion, peeled and diced
160 g root vegetables (e.g. carrot, turnip, parsnip) peeled and cut into 2.5 cm (1 in) cubes
75 g mushrooms, halved
125 ml red wine
200 ml reduced salt stock (liquid concentrate or stock cube)
2 tsp cornflour

1 Dry fry the beef in a large non-stick pan, stirring continuously until browned.

2 Add the onion and continue to cook for 2–3 minutes.

3 Add mixed root vegetables and mushrooms, and cook for a further 2–3 minutes.

4 Add the wine to the pan and allow to boil for a minute to burn off the alcohol.

5 Mix the cornflour with a little of the stock. Add to the meat and vegetable mixture and stir well.

6 Cover the meat and vegetables with the rest of the stock, bring to simmering point and put the lid on the pan.

7 Cook in a preheated oven (Gas mark 4, 180 °C) for 2–3 hours until meat is very tender.

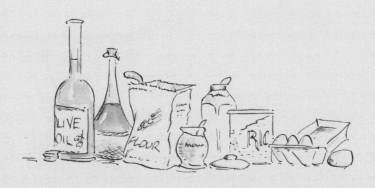

- ▶ All serving sizes are for 1 person.

- ▶ Ingredients are standard unless otherwise listed as low fat, reduced sugar, fat free etc.

- ▶ Ready-made meals or ingredients are indicated with an * asterisk.

Please note that where the GDA for sugar exceeds 90 g for the day, any extra sugars are naturally occurring sugars and not added sugar. Many foods with naturally occurring sugars are excellent sources of vitamins, minerals and fibre and these nutritional benefits outweigh the slight excess in sugar. Any excess in natural sugars has been balanced by reductions in fat so that your total calories for the day remain within the GDA.

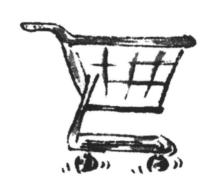

DAY 1
TOTAL GDA FOR THE DAY

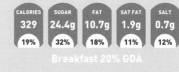

CALORIES	SUGAR	FAT	SAT FAT	SALT
1552	86.4g	48.4g	17.0g	4.0g
91%	113%	81%	100%	67%

Breakfast
125 ml fruit juice
2 slices wholegrain toast *with*
2 tsp reduced fat spread *and* 2 tsp
   jam

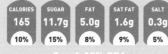

CALORIES	SUGAR	FAT	SAT FAT	SALT
329	24.4g	10.7g	1.9g	0.7g
19%	32%	18%	11%	12%

Breakfast 20% GDA

First Snack
4 small water biscuits
2 tsp low-fat soft cheese
1 apple

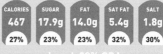

CALORIES	SUGAR	FAT	SAT FAT	SALT
165	11.7g	5.0g	1.6g	0.3g
10%	15%	8%	9%	5%

Snack 10% GDA

Lunch
1 * salmon and cucumber
   sandwich
1 × 40 g cereal and dried fruit bar

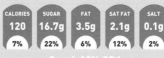

CALORIES	SUGAR	FAT	SAT FAT	SALT
467	17.9g	14.0g	5.4g	1.8g
27%	23%	23%	32%	30%

Lunch 30% GDA

Second Snack
125 g pot probiotic yogurt
handful of grapes

CALORIES	SUGAR	FAT	SAT FAT	SALT
120	16.7g	3.5g	2.1g	0.1g
7%	22%	6%	12%	2%

Snack 10% GDA

Dinner
½ a 410 g *individual margarita
   pizza with*
a large mixed salad *and*
1 tbsp fat-free dressing
Satsuma

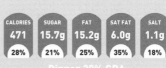

CALORIES	SUGAR	FAT	SAT FAT	SALT
471	15.7g	15.2g	6.0g	1.1g
28%	21%	25%	35%	18%

Dinner 30% GDA

1700 kcal plan FOR BUSY PEOPLE

DAY 2
TOTAL GDA FOR THE DAY

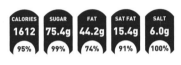

Breakfast

40 g corn flakes *with*
130 ml semi-skimmed milk
1 slice wholegrain toast *with*
1 tsp reduced-fat spread
½ grapefruit *with*
½ tsp sugar

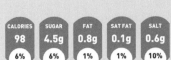

First Snack

½ (15 g) packet mini rye
  crispbread snacks

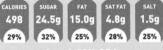

Lunch

300 g *fresh Red Thai chicken
  soup *with*
1 granary roll
60 g strawberries

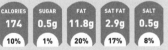

Second Snack

3 water biscuits *with*
30 g *low-fat pâté (any type)

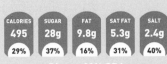

Dinner

450 g *potato-topped chicken and
  broccoli pie *with*
2 × 80 g portions vegetables (e.g.
  carrots and sweetcorn)
handful of raspberries with
  *individual meringue nest
1 tbsp low-fat natural yogurt

DAY 3
TOTAL GDA FOR THE DAY

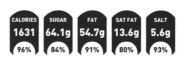

CALORIES	SUGAR	FAT	SAT FAT	SALT
1631	64.1g	54.7g	13.6g	5.6g
96%	84%	91%	80%	93%

Breakfast
80 g melon
50 g no-added-sugar muesli *with*
2 tbsp low-fat natural yogurt
1 toasted crumpet *with*
1 tsp reduced-fat spread

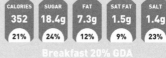

CALORIES	SUGAR	FAT	SAT FAT	SALT
352	18.4g	7.3g	1.5g	1.4g
21%	24%	12%	9%	23%

Breakfast 20% GDA

First Snack
2 tsp *chocolate and nut spread
on
1 thin slice wholegrain toast

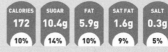

CALORIES	SUGAR	FAT	SAT FAT	SALT
172	10.4g	5.9g	1.6g	0.3g
10%	14%	10%	9%	5%

Snack 10% GDA

Lunch
1 *egg and cress sandwich
1 banana

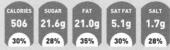

CALORIES	SUGAR	FAT	SAT FAT	SALT
506	21.6g	21.0g	5.1g	1.7g
30%	28%	35%	30%	28%

Lunch 30% GDA

Second Snack
Vegetable crudités (choose two
    from: 1 carrot, 2 stick of
    celery, 1 red pepper, 4
    broccoli florets) *with*
1 tbsp *houmous

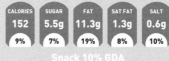

CALORIES	SUGAR	FAT	SAT FAT	SALT
152	5.5g	11.3g	1.3g	0.6g
9%	7%	19%	8%	10%

Snack 10% GDA

Dinner
400 g *spaghetti bolognese *with*
large dessert bowl of mixed
    salad *and*
1 tbsp *fat-free dressing

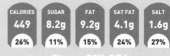

CALORIES	SUGAR	FAT	SAT FAT	SALT
449	8.2g	9.2g	4.1g	1.6g
26%	11%	15%	24%	27%

Dinner 30% GDA

DAY 4
TOTAL GDA FOR THE DAY

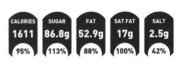

CALORIES	SUGAR	FAT	SAT FAT	SALT
1611	86.8g	52.9g	17g	2.5g
95%	113%	88%	100%	42%

Breakfast
35g ready-to-eat prunes
1 × 27g sachet instant porridge *with*
150ml semi-skimmed milk
1 slice wholegrain toast *with*
1 tsp jam

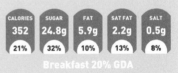

CALORIES	SUGAR	FAT	SAT FAT	SALT
352	24.8g	5.9g	2.2g	0.5g
21%	32%	10%	13%	8%

Breakfast 20% GDA

First Snack
1 × 23g cereal and dried fruit bar
80g melon

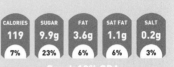

CALORIES	SUGAR	FAT	SAT FAT	SALT
119	9.9g	3.6g	1.1g	0.2g
7%	23%	6%	6%	3%

Snack 10% GDA

Lunch
1 *individual, char-grilled chicken and pasta salad
1 banana

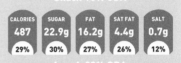

CALORIES	SUGAR	FAT	SAT FAT	SALT
487	22.9g	16.2g	4.4g	0.7g
29%	30%	27%	26%	12%

Lunch 30% GDA

Second Snack
4 water biscuits *with*
2 tsp low-fat soft cheese

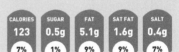

CALORIES	SUGAR	FAT	SAT FAT	SALT
123	0.5g	5.1g	1.6g	0.4g
7%	1%	9%	9%	7%

Snack 10% GDA

Dinner
100g *broccoli quiche *with*
170g boiled new potatoes *and*
2 × 80g servings of vegetables of choice *or*
a large dessert bowl of mixed salad
120g can peaches in juice *with*
1 scoop light vanilla ice-cream

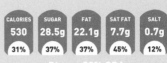

CALORIES	SUGAR	FAT	SAT FAT	SALT
530	28.5g	22.1g	7.7g	0.7g
31%	37%	37%	45%	12%

Dinner 30% GDA

DAY 5
TOTAL GDA FOR THE DAY

CALORIES	SUGAR	FAT	SAT FAT	SALT
1700	78.9g	45.1g	10.9g	6.0g
100%	103%	75%	64%	100%

Breakfast
40g puffed wheat cereal *with*
130ml semi-skimmed milk
1 toasted crumpet *with* 1 tsp jam
small handful of grapes

First Snack
1 toasted English muffin *and*
1 tsp reduced fat spread

Lunch
1 *tuna and sweetcorn sandwich
125g pot *jelly *and*
handful of fresh raspberries

Second Snack
2 *Scotch pancakes

Dinner
450g ready meal (two) sausages
and mash *with*
2 × 80g servings of vegetables of
choice
90g stewed apple *with*
1 heaped tbsp low-fat natural
yogurt

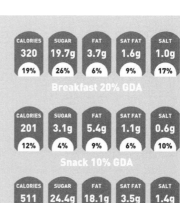

CALORIES	SUGAR	FAT	SAT FAT	SALT
320	19.7g	3.7g	1.6g	1.0g
19%	26%	6%	9%	17%

Breakfast 20% GDA

CALORIES	SUGAR	FAT	SAT FAT	SALT
201	3.1g	5.4g	1.1g	0.6g
12%	4%	9%	6%	10%

Snack 10% GDA

CALORIES	SUGAR	FAT	SAT FAT	SALT
511	24.4g	18.1g	3.5g	1.4g
30%	32%	30%	21%	23%

Lunch 30% GDA

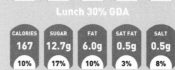

CALORIES	SUGAR	FAT	SAT FAT	SALT
167	12.7g	6.0g	0.5g	0.5g
10%	17%	10%	3%	8%

Snack 10% GDA

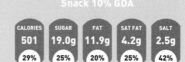

CALORIES	SUGAR	FAT	SAT FAT	SALT
501	19.0g	11.9g	4.2g	2.5g
29%	25%	20%	25%	42%

Dinner 30% GDA

DAY 6
TOTAL GDA FOR THE DAY

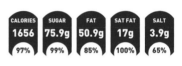

CALORIES	SUGAR	FAT	SAT FAT	SALT
1656	75.9g	50.9g	17g	3.9g
97%	99%	85%	100%	65%

Breakfast
6 sliced strawberries
2 wheat biscuits *with*
150 ml semi-skimmed milk
1 slice wholegrain toast *with*
1 tsp honey

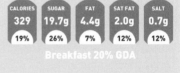

CALORIES	SUGAR	FAT	SAT FAT	SALT
329	19.7g	4.4g	2.0g	0.7g
19%	26%	7%	12%	12%

Breakfast 20% GDA

First Snack
Small bunch grapes
4 small water biscuits *with*
1 tbsp cottage cheese

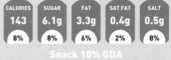

CALORIES	SUGAR	FAT	SAT FAT	SALT
143	6.1g	3.3g	0.4g	0.5g
8%	8%	6%	2%	8%

Snack 10% GDA

Lunch
1 *chicken caesar wrap
1 satsuma

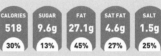

CALORIES	SUGAR	FAT	SAT FAT	SALT
518	9.6g	27.1g	4.6g	1.5g
30%	13%	45%	27%	25%

Lunch 30% GDA

Second Snack
250 ml *fruit smoothie

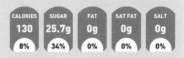

CALORIES	SUGAR	FAT	SAT FAT	SALT
130	25.7g	0g	0g	0g
8%	34%	0%	0%	0%

Snack 10% GDA

Dinner
400 g *king prawn and vegetable
   masala with rice *or*
*chicken curry *with* rice
Real strawberry milkshake *made*
   with
180 ml semi-skimmed milk *and*
2 tsp low fat yogurt *and*
8–10 strawberries, blended in a
   liquidiser

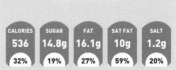

CALORIES	SUGAR	FAT	SAT FAT	SALT
536	14.8g	16.1g	10g	1.2g
32%	19%	27%	59%	20%

Dinner 30% GDA

DAY 7
TOTAL GDA FOR THE DAY

CALORIES	SUGAR	FAT	SAT FAT	SALT
151	87g	54.6g	15.8g	5.9g
94%	114%	91%	93%	98%

Breakfast
125 ml fruit juice
2 egg scrambled in a non-stick
    pan *made with* 2 tbsp semi-
    skimmed milk
2 slices wholegrain toast *with*
2 grilled tomatoes *and*
2 tbsp sliced mushrooms,
    sautéed using spray oil

CALORIES	SUGAR	FAT	SAT FAT	SALT
333	6.5g	13.5g	4.4g	1g
20%	8%	23%	26%	17%

Breakfast 20% GDA

First Snack
1 small banana, sliced *with*
1 tbsp low-fat natural yogurt *and*
1 tbsp no-added-sugar muesli

CALORIES	SUGAR	FAT	SAT FAT	SALT
147	20.0g	1.5g	0.4g	0.1g
9%	26%	3%	2%	2%

Snack 10% GDA

Lunch
300 g *fresh lentil and tomato
    soup
1 small granary roll
1 plain scone *with*
1 tsp reduced-fat spread

CALORIES	SUGAR	FAT	SAT FAT	SALT
502	15.6g	16.9g	2.9g	3g
30%	20%	28%	17%	50%

Lunch 30% GDA

Second Snack
2 fingers Kit Kat
1 apple

CALORIES	SUGAR	FAT	SAT FAT	SALT
141	18.0g	5.8g	3.6g	0.7g
8%	24%	10%	21%	12%

Snack 10% GDA

Dinner
2 slices roast beef with gravy
    (from oven-ready roasting
    joint)
2 scoops mashed potato (fresh or
    instant)
2 × 80 g portions of vegetables
75 g *fruit crumble *and*
2 tsp low-fat yoghurt

CALORIES	SUGAR	FAT	SAT FAT	SALT
468	26.9g	16.9g	4.5g	1.1g
28%	35%	28%	26%	18%

Dinner 30% GDA

- ▶ All serving sizes are for 1 person.

- ▶ Ingredients are standard unless otherwise listed as low fat, reduced sugar, fat free etc.

- ▶ Ready-made meals or ingredients are indicated with an * asterisk. Meals where recipes are provided are indicated in **bold**.

Please note that where the GDA for sugar exceeds 90g for the day, any extra sugars are naturally occurring sugars and not added sugar. Many foods with naturally occurring sugars are excellent sources of vitamins, minerals and fibre and these nutritional benefits outweigh the slight excess in sugar. Any excess in natural sugars has been balanced by reductions in fat so that your total calories for the day remain within the GDA.

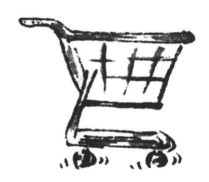

DAY 1
TOTAL GDA FOR THE DAY

CALORIES	SUGAR	FAT	SAT FAT	SALT
1628	75.9g	59.5g	14.5g	5.5g
96%	99%	99%	85%	92%

Breakfast
½ grapefruit *with* 1 tsp sugar
1 low-fat croissant
1 slice wholemeal toast *with*
2 tsp jam

CALORIES	SUGAR	FAT	SAT FAT	SALT
309	23.9g	7.6g	3.8g	0.7g
18%	31%	13%	22%	12%

Breakfast 20% GDA

First Snack
250 ml *mango and strawberry
    smoothie

CALORIES	SUGAR	FAT	SAT FAT	SALT
158	20.9g	5.8g	3.7g	0.1g
9%	27%	10%	22%	2%

Snack 10% GDA

Lunch
300 g *mixed bean and tomato
    soup
1 small granary roll
1 toasted teacake *with*
1 tsp reduced-fat spread

CALORIES	SUGAR	FAT	SAT FAT	SALT
508	21.5g	11.5g	2.7g	2.4g
30%	28%	19%	16%	40%

Lunch 30% GDA

Second Snack
Vegetable crudités (use 2 of the
    following: 1 carrot, 1 red
    pepper, 2 celery sticks, 4–5
    broccoli florets)
with 1 tbsp *houmous

CALORIES	SUGAR	FAT	SAT FAT	SALT
152	5.5g	10.9g	1.3g	0.6g
9%	7%	18%	8%	10%

Snack 10% GDA

Dinner
1 × nutty chickpea burger *with*
1 pitta bread
A large dessert bowl of mixed
    salad *with*
2 tsp *fat-free dressing

CALORIES	SUGAR	FAT	SAT FAT	SALT
501	4.1g	23.7g	3.0g	1.7g
29%	5%	40%	18%	28%

Dinner 30% GDA

RECIPE
Nutty chickpea burgers
See page 92.

DAY 2
TOTAL GDA FOR THE DAY

CALORIES	SUGAR	FAT	SAT FAT	SALT
1593	84.5g	52g	17g	6.0g
94%	110%	87%	100%	100%

Breakfast
40 g puffed wheat cereal *with*
130 ml semi-skimmed milk *and*
handful of blueberries
1 toasted crumpet *with* 1 tsp
    reduced fat spread

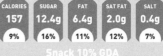

CALORIES	SUGAR	FAT	SAT FAT	SALT
356	14.6g	7g	1.7g	1.0g
21%	19%	12%	10%	17%

Breakfast 20% GDA

First Snack
1 tbsp *guacamole
3 breadsticks
1 apple

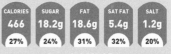

CALORIES	SUGAR	FAT	SAT FAT	SALT
157	12.4g	6.4g	2.0g	0.4g
9%	16%	11%	12%	7%

Snack 10% GDA

Lunch
1 *egg and salad sandwich on
    wholemeal bread
1 × 23 g dried fruit and cereal bar
1 peach or nectarine

CALORIES	SUGAR	FAT	SAT FAT	SALT
466	18.2g	18.6g	5.4g	1.2g
27%	24%	31%	32%	20%

Lunch 30% GDA

Second Snack
3 water biscuits *with* 1 tsp jam
    and
1 tbsp peanut butter

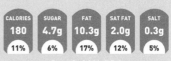

CALORIES	SUGAR	FAT	SAT FAT	SALT
180	4.7g	10.3g	2.0g	0.3g
11%	6%	17%	12%	5%

Snack 10% GDA

Dinner
350 g *vegetable lasagne
a large dessert bowl of mixed
    salad *and*
1 tbsp *fat-free dressing
100 g fruit salad *and*
1 tbsp low-fat yogurt

CALORIES	SUGAR	FAT	SAT FAT	SALT
434	34.6g	9.7g	5.9g	3.1g
26%	45%	16%	35%	52%

Dinner 30% GDA

DAY 3
TOTAL GDA FOR THE DAY

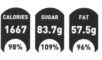

CALORIES	SUGAR	FAT	SAT FAT	SALT
1667	83.7g	57.5g	16.8g	5g
98%	109%	96%	99%	83%

Breakfast
2 wheat biscuits *with*
130 ml semi-skimmed milk
1 slice wholegrain toast *with*
1 tsp reduced fat spread
handful of sliced strawberries

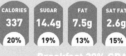

CALORIES	SUGAR	FAT	SAT FAT	SALT
337	14.4g	7.5g	2.6g	0.8g
20%	19%	13%	15%	13%

Breakfast 20% GDA

First Snack
Avocado and tomato salad

CALORIES	SUGAR	FAT	SAT FAT	SALT
173	4.2g	14.5g	2.6g	0.1g
10%	5%	24%	15%	2%

Snack 10% GDA

Lunch
90 g wholemeal pitta bread *filled with*
Greek salad *and*
1 tsp *fat-free dressing
1 sliced banana *with*
2 tbsp low-fat yogurt *and*
1 tbsp granola

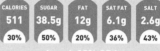

CALORIES	SUGAR	FAT	SAT FAT	SALT
511	38.5g	12g	6.1g	2.6g
30%	50%	20%	36%	43%

Lunch 30% GDA

Second Snack
1 tsp chocolate and nut spread
1 thin slice wholegrain toast

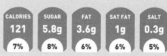

CALORIES	SUGAR	FAT	SAT FAT	SALT
121	5.8g	3.6g	1g	0.3g
7%	8%	6%	6%	5%

Snack 10% GDA

Dinner
100 g *broccoli, tomato and cheese quiche *with*
170 g boiled new potatoes *and*
2 × 80 g portions of vegetables of choice *or*
a large dessert bowl of mixed salad
2 *Scotch pancakes

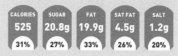

CALORIES	SUGAR	FAT	SAT FAT	SALT
525	20.8g	19.9g	4.5g	1.2g
31%	27%	33%	26%	20%

Dinner 30% GDA

RECIPES
Greek salad
See recipe on page 95, but use only 40 g of feta cheese.
Avocado and tomato salad
See recipe on page 95.

DAY 4
TOTAL GDA FOR THE DAY

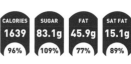

CALORIES	SUGAR	FAT	SAT FAT	SALT
1639	83.1g	45.9g	15.1g	6.0g
96%	109%	77%	89%	100%

Breakfast
40 g corn flakes *with*
130 ml semi-skimmed milk
1 slice wholegrain toast *with*
1 tsp reduced-fat spread
½ grapefruit *with* 1 tsp sugar

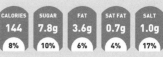

CALORIES	SUGAR	FAT	SAT FAT	SALT
347	17.9g	6.8g	2.3g	1.1g
20%	23%	11%	14%	18%

Breakfast 20% GDA

First Snack
150 g melon
1 toasted crumpet *with*
1 tsp reduced-fat spread

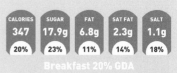

CALORIES	SUGAR	FAT	SAT FAT	SALT
144	7.8g	3.6g	0.7g	1.0g
8%	10%	6%	4%	17%

Snack 10% GDA

Lunch
1 small tin (210 g) baked beans
   (reduced sugar and salt
   variety), heated *on*
2 slices wholemeal toast *with*
2 tsp reduced-fat spread
1 tbsp low-fat yogurt *with*
2 tbsp no-added-sugar muesli
   and
1 sliced banana

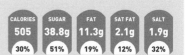

CALORIES	SUGAR	FAT	SAT FAT	SALT
505	38.8g	11.3g	2.1g	1.9g
30%	51%	19%	12%	32%

Lunch 30% GDA

Second Snack
4 water biscuits *with*
40 g *mushroom pâté

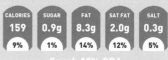

CALORIES	SUGAR	FAT	SAT FAT	SALT
159	0.9g	8.3g	2.0g	0.3g
9%	1%	14%	12%	5%

Snack 10% GDA

Dinner
**Broad bean, beetroot and goats
   cheese salad** *with*
1 wholemeal pitta bread
1 kiwi fruit

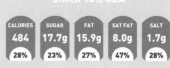

CALORIES	SUGAR	FAT	SAT FAT	SALT
484	17.7g	15.9g	8.0g	1.7g
28%	23%	27%	47%	28%

Dinner 30% GDA

RECIPE
**Broad bean, beetroot and goats
   cheese salad**
See recipe on page 97.

DAY 5
TOTAL GDA FOR THE DAY

CALORIES	SUGAR	FAT	SAT FAT	SALT
1600	87.1g	52.9g	9.0g	6.0g
94%	114%	88%	53%	100%

Breakfast
50 g no-added-sugar muesli
2 tbsp low-fat natural yogurt
1 slice wholemeal toast *with*
1 tsp reduced-fat spread

CALORIES	SUGAR	FAT	SAT FAT	SALT
333	14.2g	8.8g	2.0g	0.5g
20%	19%	15%	12%	8%

Breakfast 20% GDA

First Snack
4 water biscuits
1 tbsp cottage cheese
Small bunch grapes

CALORIES	SUGAR	FAT	SAT FAT	SALT
164	9.0g	4.3g	0.9g	0.5g
10%	12%	7%	5%	8%

Snack 10% GDA

Lunch
**Roasted vegetable and reduced-
fat houmous wrap (100 g
mixed roasted vegetables)**
1 tbsp natural yogurt *with*
1 tbsp granola *and*
1 small banana

CALORIES	SUGAR	FAT	SAT FAT	SALT
430	24.9g	19.1g	3.8g	2.2g
25%	33%	32%	22%	37%

Lunch 30% GDA

Second Snack
10 almonds *and*
4 dried apricots

CALORIES	SUGAR	FAT	SAT FAT	SALT
189	14.1g	11.9g	0.9g	0.1g
11%	18%	20%	5%	2%

Snack 10% GDA

Dinner
**Spaghetti bolognese with
Quorn™ mince**
with a large mixed salad *and*
1 tbsp *fat-free dressing
1 large orange

CALORIES	SUGAR	FAT	SAT FAT	SALT
484	24.9g	8.8g	1.4g	2.7g
28%	33%	15%	8%	45%

Dinner 30% GDA

RECIPES
Roasted vegetable wrap
*See recipe on page 99, but use
low-fat houmous.*
**Spaghetti bolognese with Quorn
mince**
See recipe on page 99.

DAY 6
TOTAL GDA FOR THE DAY

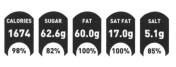

CALORIES	SUGAR	FAT	SAT FAT	SALT
1674	62.6g	60.0g	17.0g	5.1g
98%	82%	100%	100%	85%

Breakfast
125 ml fruit juice
1 egg scrambled in non-stick pan *with*
2 tbsp semi-skimmed milk
2 slices wholegrain toast *with*
2 grilled tomatoes *and*
2 tbsp sliced mushrooms, sautéed using spray oil

CALORIES	SUGAR	FAT	SAT FAT	SALT
405	18.5g	14.9g	4.2g	0.8g
240%	24%	25%	25%	13%

Breakfast 20% GDA

First Snack
Individual lentil and tomato salad

CALORIES	SUGAR	FAT	SAT FAT	SALT
158	3.5g	6.5g	0.8g	0.8g
9%	5%	11%	5%	13%

Snack 10% GDA

Lunch
Vegetarian niçoise salad *with*
5 cm (2 in) baguette
1 toasted teacake *and*
2 tsp reduced-fat spread

CALORIES	SUGAR	FAT	SAT FAT	SALT
494	15.7g	19.3g	5.1g	1.6g
29%	21%	32%	30%	27%

Lunch 30% GDA

Second Snack
1 tbsp *tzatziki *with*
Vegetable crudités (choose two from: 1 carrot, 1 yellow pepper, 4 broccoli florets, 2 celery sticks)
4 breadsticks

CALORIES	SUGAR	FAT	SAT FAT	SALT
139	7.9g	4.0g	1.0g	0.8g
8%	10%	7%	6%	13%

Snack 10% GDA

Dinner
½ *margarita pizza (410 g) *with*
large dessert bowl of mixed salad *and*
1 tbsp *fat-free dressing
1 satsuma

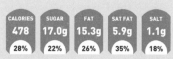

CALORIES	SUGAR	FAT	SAT FAT	SALT
478	17.0g	15.3g	5.9g	1.1g
28%	22%	26%	35%	18%

Dinner 30% GDA

RECIPES
Vegetarian niçoise salad
See recipe on page 101.
Individual lentil and tomato salad
See recipe on page 101.

DAY 7
TOTAL GDA FOR THE DAY

CALORIES	SUGAR	FAT	SAT FAT	SALT
1598	75.0g	56.8g	15.2g	5.9g
94%	98%	95%	89%	98%

Breakfast
Porridge *made with* 50 g oats *and*
240 ml semi-skimmed milk
   topped with
1 tbsp raisins tossed in 1 tsp
   ground cinnamon

CALORIES	SUGAR	FAT	SAT FAT	SALT
319	19.4g	8.1g	3.2g	0.2g
19%	25%	14%	19%	3%

Breakfast 20% GDA

First Snack
4 water biscuits *with*
1 tbsp low-fat soft cheese
handful of grapes

CALORIES	SUGAR	FAT	SAT FAT	SALT
151	7.3g	4.0g	2.2g	0.6g
9%	10%	7%	13%	10%

Snack 10% GDA

Lunch
**Spinach, feta cheese and
   mushroom omelette** *with* a
   large mixed salad *and*
1 tbsp low-fat vinaigrette (page
   169) *and*
1 large wholemeal roll
1 apple

CALORIES	SUGAR	FAT	SAT FAT	SALT
462	16.7g	22.5g	7.3g	2.4g
27%	22%	38%	43%	40%

Lunch 30% GDA

Second Snack
1 slice wholemeal toast *with*
1 tsp jam and 1 tsp peanut butter

CALORIES	SUGAR	FAT	SAT FAT	SALT
168	7.2g	6.9g	1.2g	0.4g
10%	9%	12%	7%	7%

Snack 10% GDA

Dinner
**Falafel and lemon couscous with
   a tomato salad** *with*
5 cm (2 in) chunk of crusty bread
120 g fruit salad

CALORIES	SUGAR	FAT	SAT FAT	SALT
498	24.4g	15.3g	1.3g	2.3g
29%	32%	26%	8%	38%

Dinner 30% GDA

RECIPES
**Spinach, feta and mushroom
   omelette**
See recipe on page 103.
**Falafel and lemon couscous with
   a tomato salad**
See recipe on page 103.

► All serving sizes are for 1 person.

► Ingredients are standard unless otherwise listed as low fat, reduced sugar, fat free etc.

► Ready-made meals or ingredients are listed with an * asterisk. Meals where recipes are provided are indicated in **bold**.

Please note that where the GDA for sugar exceeds 90 g for the day, any extra sugars are naturally occurring sugars and not added sugar. Many foods with naturally occurring sugars are excellent sources of vitamins, minerals and fibre and these nutritional benefits outweigh the slight excess in sugar. Any excess in natural sugars has been balanced by reductions in fat so that your total calories for the day remain within the GDA.

Average portion sizes are included in savvy GDA tips (see page 177).

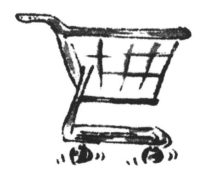

DAY 1
TOTAL GDA FOR THE DAY

CALORIES	SUGAR	FAT	SAT FAT	SALT
1556	69.7g	46.8g	17g	6.0g
92%	91%	78%	100%	100%

Breakfast
80g grapefruit segments in light syrup
50g cornflakes *with*
135ml semi-skimmed milk
1 slice wholemeal toast *with*
1tsp reduced-fat spread

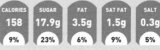

CALORIES	SUGAR	FAT	SAT FAT	SALT
382	22.8g	6.0g	2.2g	1.5g
22%	30%	10%	13%	25%

Breakfast 20% GDA

First Snack
1 digestive
1 × 125g low-fat fruit yogurt

CALORIES	SUGAR	FAT	SAT FAT	SALT
158	17.9g	3.5g	1.5g	0.3g
9%	23%	6%	9%	5%

Snack 10% GDA

Lunch
Home made tuna and sweetcorn sandwich on wholemeal bread
1 *Scotch pancake
handful of grapes

CALORIES	SUGAR	FAT	SAT FAT	SALT
426	16.9g	12g	2.8g	1.4g
25%	22%	20%	16%	23%

Lunch 30% GDA

Second Snack
4 water biscuits *with*
30g *low-fat pâté

CALORIES	SUGAR	FAT	SAT FAT	SALT
178	0.6g	10.1g	2.5g	0.7g
10%	1%	17%	15%	12%

Snack 10% GDA

Dinner
300g *meat or vegetable lasagne *with*
a large dessert bowl of mixed salad *and* 1tbsp *fat-free dressing
handful of grapes

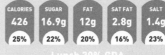
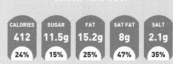

CALORIES	SUGAR	FAT	SAT FAT	SALT
412	11.5g	15.2g	8g	2.1g
24%	15%	25%	47%	35%

Dinner 30% GDA

1700 kcal plan ON A BUDGET

DAY 2
TOTAL GDA FOR THE DAY

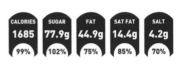

CALORIES	SUGAR	FAT	SAT FAT	SALT
1685	77.9g	44.9g	14.4g	4.2g
99%	102%	75%	85%	70%

Breakfast
3 tbsp muesli *with*
140 ml semi-skimmed milk
125 ml breakfast juice
1 slice wholemeal toast *with*
1 tsp reduced-fat spread *and*
1 tsp jam

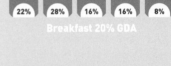

CALORIES	SUGAR	FAT	SAT FAT	SALT
382	21.7g	9.3g	2.7g	0.5g
22%	28%	16%	16%	8%

Breakfast 20% GDA

First Snack
1 scotch pancake
1 pear

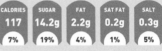

CALORIES	SUGAR	FAT	SAT FAT	SALT
117	14.2g	2.2g	0.2g	0.3g
7%	19%	4%	1%	5%

Snack 10% GDA

Lunch
1 medium baked potato *with*
1 small tin (200 g) baked beans,
    heated *and*
20 g grated cheese

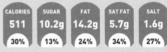

CALORIES	SUGAR	FAT	SAT FAT	SALT
511	10.2g	14.2g	5.7g	1.6g
30%	13%	24%	34%	27%

Lunch 30% GDA

Second Snack
2 tbsp natural yogurt *and*
2 tbsp oats *with*
1 small banana, sliced

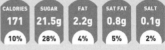

CALORIES	SUGAR	FAT	SAT FAT	SALT
171	21.5g	2.2g	0.8g	0.1g
10%	28%	4%	5%	2%

Snack 10% GDA

Dinner
1 medium pork chop, grilled
2 scoops mashed potato *and*
2 × 80 g servings of vegetables
    with
45 g gravy 168
1 *Scotch pancake

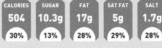

CALORIES	SUGAR	FAT	SAT FAT	SALT
504	10.3g	17g	5g	1.7g
30%	13%	28%	29%	28%

Dinner 30% GDA

DAY 3
TOTAL GDA FOR THE DAY

CALORIES	SUGAR	FAT	SAT FAT	SALT
1625	80.1g	46.9g	15.0g	5.1g
96%	105%	78%	88%	85%

1700 kcal plan ON A BUDGET

Breakfast
30g rice krispies *with*
140ml semi-skimmed milk
½ grapefruit *with* 1 tsp sugar
1 slice wholemeal toast *with*
1 tsp reduced-fat spread *and*
scraping of yeast extract

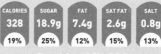

CALORIES	SUGAR	FAT	SAT FAT	SALT
328	18.9g	7.4g	2.6g	0.8g
19%	25%	12%	15%	13%

Breakfast 20% GDA

First Snack
1 *sultana scone *with*
1 tsp reduced-fat spread

CALORIES	SUGAR	FAT	SAT FAT	SALT
161	4.4g	7.0g	2.0g	0.6g
9%	6%	12%	12%	10%

Snack 10% GDA

Lunch
½ 200g can tomato soup *with*
1 wholemeal roll
1 toasted teacake *with*
1 tsp reduced-fat spread
1 apple

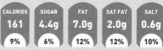

CALORIES	SUGAR	FAT	SAT FAT	SALT
497	30.0g	11.3g	2.6g	2.6g
29%	39%	19%	15%	43%

Lunch 30% GDA

Second Snack
3 water biscuits *with*
1 tbsp plain cottage cheese
small handful of grapes

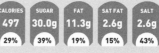

CALORIES	SUGAR	FAT	SAT FAT	SALT
134	7.8g	3.6g	0.9g	0.4g
8%	10%	6%	5%	7%

Snack 10% GDA

Dinner
¼ (75g) *cheese and bacon
    quiche *with*
180g (6) new potatoes, boiled *and*
a large dessert bowl of mixed
    salad *or*
2 × 80g portions of vegetables
140g stewed fruit *with*
2 tbsp *low-fat custard

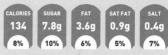

CALORIES	SUGAR	FAT	SAT FAT	SALT
505	19.0g	17.6g	6.9g	0.7g
30%	25%	29%	41%	12%

Dinner 30% GDA

DAY 4
TOTAL GDA FOR THE DAY

CALORIES	SUGAR	FAT	SAT FAT	SALT
1626	84.7g	57.7g	15.1g	5.2g
96%	111%	96%	89%	87%

Breakfast
3 wheat biscuits *with*
150 ml semi-skimmed milk
    topped with sliced apple
1 slice wholemeal toast
with 1 tsp honey

CALORIES	SUGAR	FAT	SAT FAT	SALT
360	22.4g	4.7g	1.9g	0.7g
21%	29%	8%	11%	12%

Breakfast 20% GDA

First Snack
Vegetable crudités (choose two
    from: 1 carrot, 1 yellow
    pepper, 4 broccoli florets,
    2 celery sticks) *with*
1 tbsp *houmous

CALORIES	SUGAR	FAT	SAT FAT	SALT
179	5.1g	13.8g	0.1g	0.3g
11%	7%	23%	0.6%	5%

Snack 10% GDA

Lunch
Home-made sandwich on
    wholemeal bread made *with*
1 slice ham and 25 g cheese, *with*
1 sliced tomato and handful of
    lettuce, *with* 1 tsp low-calorie
    mayonnaise
100 g can peaches in light syrup
    with
1 tbsp low-fat yogurt

CALORIES	SUGAR	FAT	SAT FAT	SALT
445	24.4g	17g	6.7g	2.4g
26%	32%	28%	39%	40%

Lunch 30% GDA

Second Snack
2 Jaffa cakes *with*
1 mug instant low-calorie hot
    chocolate

CALORIES	SUGAR	FAT	SAT FAT	SALT
164	24.3g	4.3g	3.2g	0.2g
10%	32%	7%	19%	3%

Snack 10% GDA

Dinner
Pasta bolognese *with*
a large dessert bowl of mixed
    salad *and*
1 tbsp fat-free dressing

CALORIES	SUGAR	FAT	SAT FAT	SALT
478	8.5g	17.9g	3.2g	1.6g
28%	11%	30%	19%	27%

Dinner 30% GDA

DAY 4 RECIPE

Pasta bolognese

The same recipe as page 111, but with reduced quantities.

70 g turkey or pork mince, raw
½ onion, diced
Handful of mushrooms, sliced
100 g jar bolognese sauce
50 g (dry weight) spaghetti or pasta shapes

1 Dry fry the mince in a non-stick pan, stirring all the time until it begins to brown.

2 Add the onion and mushrooms and continue to stir, cook for 6–7 minutes until softened.

3 Add bolognese sauce and simmer gently for 10 minutes.

4 Cook the pasta according to packet instructions.

Serve cooked bolognese on a bed of pasta.

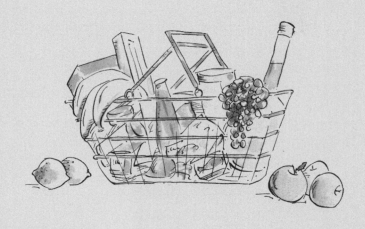

DAY 5
TOTAL GDA FOR THE DAY

CALORIES	SUGAR	FAT	SAT FAT	SALT
1647	82g	46.6g	13.7g	6.0g
97%	107%	78%	81%	100%

Breakfast
125 ml orange juice
2 slices wholemeal toast *with*
2 tsp reduced-fat spread *and*
2 tsp jam

CALORIES	SUGAR	FAT	SAT FAT	SALT
305	26.0g	7.6g	2.4g	0.7g
18%	34%	13%	14%	12%

Breakfast 20% GDA

First Snack
Large handful of grapes
4 water biscuits *topped with*
30 g reduced-fat cream cheese

CALORIES	SUGAR	FAT	SAT FAT	SALT
142	4.9g	4.2g	1.0g	0.5g
8%	6%	7%	6%	8%

Snack 10% GDA

Lunch
100 g canned mackerel *with*
100 g (dry weight) pasta shells,
   cooked
a large dessert bowl of mixed
   salad *and*
1 tbsp *fat-free dressing plus
125 g pot low-fat yogurt

CALORIES	SUGAR	FAT	SAT FAT	SALT
520	22.0g	20.3g	4.8g	1.3g
31%	29%	34%	28%	22%

Lunch 30% GDA

Second Snack
2 toasted crumpets *with*
2 tsp jam

CALORIES	SUGAR	FAT	SAT FAT	SALT
171	11.5g	0.6g	0.1g	1.1g
10%	15%	1%	%	18%

Snack 10% GDA

Dinner
1 individual *margarita pizza (or
   190 g slice from large
   margarita pizza) *with*
80 g vegetables as extra toppings
   (e.g. sliced peppers, onion,
   mushrooms) *and*
large dessert bowl of green salad
   and
1 tbsp *fat-free dressing

CALORIES	SUGAR	FAT	SAT FAT	SALT
509	17.6g	13.9g	5.4g	2.4g
30%	23%	23%	32%	40%

Dinner 30% GDA

DAY 6
TOTAL GDA FOR THE DAY

CALORIES	SUGAR	FAT	SAT FAT	SALT
1680	78.7g	59g	14g	5.9g
99%	103%	98%	82%	98%

Breakfast
1 toasted English muffin *with*
1 egg, scrambled in non-stick pan with no added butter or milk *and*
2 tbsp baked beans heated
125 ml orange juice

CALORIES	SUGAR	FAT	SAT FAT	SALT
368	19.0g	7.7g	1.9g	1.5g
22%	25%	13%	11%	25%

Breakfast 20% GDA

First Snack
2 tbsp natural yogurt *and* 2 tbsp oats *with*
1 small banana, sliced

CALORIES	SUGAR	FAT	SAT FAT	SALT
171	21.5g	2.2g	0.8g	0.1g
10%	28%	4%	5%	2%

Snack 10% GDA

Lunch
1 *vegetarian burger, grilled wholemeal bap *with*
1 tbsp *tomato salsa or chutney *and*
2 thin slices (30 g) cheese
a large dessert bowl of mixed salad *and*
1 tbsp *fat-free dressing
1 × 23 g oat and fruit cereal bar

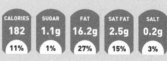

CALORIES	SUGAR	FAT	SAT FAT	SALT
501	22.8g	16.9g	7.7g	2.6g
29%	30%	28%	45%	43%

Lunch 30% GDA

Second Snack
30 g mixed unsalted nuts

CALORIES	SUGAR	FAT	SAT FAT	SALT
182	1.1g	16.2g	2.5g	0.2g
11%	1%	27%	15%	3%

Snack 10% GDA

Dinner
Chicken and vegetable stir fry.

 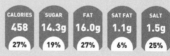

CALORIES	SUGAR	FAT	SAT FAT	SALT
458	14.3g	16.0g	1.1g	1.5g
27%	19%	27%	6%	25%

Dinner 30% GDA

RECIPE
Chicken and vegetable stir fry
See recipe on page 109.

DAY 7
TOTAL GDA FOR THE DAY

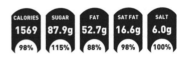

CALORIES	SUGAR	FAT	SAT FAT	SALT
1569	87.9g	52.7g	16.6g	6.0g
98%	115%	88%	98%	100%

Breakfast
1 low-fat croissant *with*
1 tsp reduced fat spread
1 toasted crumpet *with*
1 tsp reduced-fat spread
80 g canned grapefruit segments
    in light syrup

CALORIES	SUGAR	FAT	SAT FAT	SALT
311	16.2g	11.7g	5.5g	1.0g
18%	21%	20%	32%	17%

Breakfast 20% GDA

First Snack
30 g cornflakes *with*
125 ml semi-skimmed milk
Small handful of grapes

CALORIES	SUGAR	FAT	SAT FAT	SALT
187	11.7g	2.5g	1.2g	0.7g
11%	15%	4%	7%	12%

Snack 10% GDA

Lunch
200 g *tomato soup *with*
a large wholemeal roll
1 small banana, sliced *with*
2 tbsp plain low-fat yogurt

CALORIES	SUGAR	FAT	SAT FAT	SALT
384	30g	7.7g	1.7g	2.2g
23%	39%	13%	10%	37%

Lunch 30% GDA

Second Snack
2 *Scotch pancakes

CALORIES	SUGAR	FAT	SAT FAT	SALT
153	9.0g	4.2g	0.4g	0.7g
9%	12%	7%	2%	12%

Snack 10% GDA

Dinner
350 g *cottage pie *with*
2–3 80 g portions steamed
    vegetables
1 apple

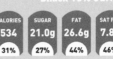

CALORIES	SUGAR	FAT	SAT FAT	SALT
534	21.0g	26.6g	7.8g	1.4g
31%	27%	44%	46%	23%

Dinner 30% GDA

THE MEAL PLANNERS

The meal planners are a combination of quick and easy meals and snacks as well as pre-prepared meals and snacks that you can find in your usual supermarket or high-street shop. See page 226 for a list of all retailers and manufacturers that currently use GDA labelling on their products. The GDA Diet website will keep you up to date with the latest additions: www.gdadiet.com.

If you have decided to follow one or more of the 7-day plans for the first couple of weeks of your GDA Diet, these food lists will be really helpful when you come to start constructing your own eating plans.

If there are any meal suggestions in the 7-day eating plans that you just don't fancy, then simply swap them for another suggestion from the meal-by-meal food lists and you can be sure that you'll be staying on track.

► In the food lists, ready-made meals or ingredients are indicated with an * asterisk.
► Meals where recipes are provided (at the end of the chapter) are indicated in **bold**.

Please note that where the GDA for sugar exceeds 90 g for the day, any extra sugars are naturally occurring sugars and not added sugar. Many foods with naturally occurring sugars are excellent sources of vitamins, minerals and fibre and these nutritional benefits outweigh the slight excess in sugar. Any excess in natural sugars has been balanced by reductions in fat so that your total calories for the day remain within the GDA.

BREAKFAST PLANNER

Breakfast 20% GDA	Calories	Sugar	Fat	Saturates	Salt
GDA target	400	18	14	4	1.2

40 g bran flakes *with*
140 ml semi-skimmed milk *with*
6 sliced strawberries
1 slices wholemeal toast *with*
1 tsp reduced-fat spread

CALORIES	SUGAR	FAT	SATURATES	SALT
335	**19.2g**	**9.7g**	**3.8g**	**1.0g**
17%	21%	14%	19%	17%

40 g corn flakes *with*
130 ml semi-skimmed milk
1 toasted English muffin *with*
1 tsp reduced-fat spread

CALORIES	SUGAR	FAT	SATURATES	SALT
382	**14.8g**	**8.0g**	**2.6g**	**1.2g**
19%	16%	11%	13%	20%

45 g mini shredded wheat *with*
150 ml semi-skimmed milk
1 slice wholemeal toast *with*
  1 tsp each jam and peanut
  butter

CALORIES	SUGAR	FAT	SATURATES	SALT
397	**14.4g**	**11.1g**	**3.4g**	**0.5g**
20%	16%	16%	17%	8%

2 slices wholemeal toast
1 tsp reduced-fat spread *with*
1 egg, scrambled in a non-stick
  pan with no added butter or
  milk, *and*
20 g smoked salmon
125 ml orange juice

CALORIES	SUGAR	FAT	SATURATES	SALT
337	**13.8g**	**14.0g**	**4.0g**	**1.5g**
17%	15%	20%	20%	25%

40 g fruit 'n fibre cereal *with*
140 ml semi-skimmed milk
1 slices wholemeal toast *with*
1 tsp reduced-fat spread

CALORIES	SUGAR	FAT	SATURATES	SALT
377	**19g**	**10.7g**	**3.3g**	**0.9g**
19%	21%	15%	17%	15%

1 toasted bagel *with* 1 tsp jam
  and 1 heaped tsp peanut
  butter
125 ml orange juice

CALORIES	SUGAR	FAT	SATURATES	SALT
336	**17.2g**	**11.8g**	**1.5g**	**1.2g**
17%	19%	17%	8%	20%

1 toasted muffin *with* 1 tsp
  reduced-fat spread *topped*
  with ½ tin (200 g) (reduced
  sugar and salt) baked beans,
  heated plus 1 grilled tomato
  and 5 sliced mushrooms
  fried in ½ tsp vegetable oil. 1
  apple

CALORIES	SUGAR	FAT	SATURATES	SALT
375	**20.1g**	**12.8g**	**3.0g**	**1.7g**
19%	22%	18%	15%	28%

(continued)

Breakfast 20% GDA	Calories	Sugar	Fat	Saturates	Salt
GDA target	400	18	14	4	1.2
40 g puffed wheat cereal and 1 pot fruit yogurt, 1 slice wholemeal toast *with* 1 tsp reduced-fat spread	CALORIES 390 20%	SUGAR 22.2g 25%	FAT 9.0g 13%	SATURATES 3.4g 17%	SALT 0.5g 8%
Porridge *made with* 60 g oats and 250 ml semi-skimmed milk *and* 2 chopped dried apricots *and* 1 tsp flaked almonds	CALORIES 391 20%	SUGAR 17.7g 20%	FAT 12.5g 18%	SATURATES 3.8g 19%	SALT 0.2g 3%
60 g muesli *with* 175 ml semi-skimmed milk 1 toasted crumpet *with* reduced-fat spread	CALORIES 393 20%	SUGAR 16.4g 18%	FAT 9.5g 14%	SATURATES 3.6g 18%	SALT 0.8g 13%

BREAKFAST PLANNER

Breakfast 20% GDA	Calories	Sugar	Fat	Saturates	Salt
GDA target	340	15.3	12	3.4	1.2

	CALORIES	SUGAR	FAT	SATURATES	SALT
1 toasted English muffin *topped with* 2 eggs, scrambled or poached plus 1 large grilled tomato	**337** 20%	**5.9g** 8%	**13.4g** 22%	**4.5g** 26%	**0.9g** 15%
2 slices wholemeal toast *topped with* 2 tsp reduced-fat spread and ½ large tin reduced sugar and salt baked beans, heated 1 pear	**333** 20%	**23.6g** 31%	**8.9g** 15%	**1.4g** 8%	**1.7g** 28%
50 g puffed wheat cereal and 150 ml semi-skimmed milk *with* 1 small banana	**331** 19%	**24.1g** 32%	**4.3g** 8%	**1.9g** 11%	**0.18g** 3%
1 boiled egg *with* toast soldiers (2 slices wholemeal bread) 2 tsp reduced-fat spread 80 g canned prunes in fruit juice	**335** 20%	**17.0g** 22%	**11.9g** 20%	**3.7g** 22%	**1.0g** 17%
2 wheat biscuits *with* 130 ml semi-skimmed milk 80 g melon 1 slice wholemeal toast *with* 1 tsp jam	**300** 18%	**21.5g** 28%	**4.0g** 7%	**1.7g** 10%	**0.6g** 10%
60 g no-added-sugar muesli *with* 2 tbsp low-fat natural yogurt 1 apple 1 kiwi fruit	**328** 19%	**25.4g** 33%	**5.0g** 8%	**1.2g** 7%	**0.1g** 2%
40 g malted square cereal *with* 130 ml semi-skimmed milk ½ grapefruit 1 toasted crumpet *with* 1 tsp reduced-fat spread	**340** 20%	**19.0g** 25%	**6.5g** 11%	**2.2g** 13%	**1.4g** 23%

(continued)

Breakfast 20% GDA	Calories	Sugar	Fat	Saturates	Salt
GDA target	340	15.3	12	3.4	1.2
Porridge (45 g oats plus 220 ml semi-skimmed milk) *with* sprinkle of ground cinnamon and 35 g ready-to-eat prunes	**CALORIES** 312 18%	**SUGAR** 21.9g 29%	**FAT** 7.6g 13%	**SATURATES** 2.9g 17%	**SALT** 0.3g 5%
2 slices wholemeal toast *topped with* 6 mushrooms and 2 tomatoes, fried gently in 1 tsp vegetable oil	**CALORIES** 305 18%	**SUGAR** 6.7g 9%	**FAT** 15.3g 26%	**SATURATES** 2.1g 12%	**SALT** 0.7g 12%
Mushroom and ham omelette *with* 2 eggs and 3 tbsp semi-skimmed milk cooked in 1 tsp vegetable oil. 1 slice wholemeal bread	**CALORIES** 322 19%	**SUGAR** X.XXg 3.34%	**FAT** 18.5g 31%	**SATURATES** 5.0g 29%	**SALT** 1.3g 22%

LUNCH PLANNER

Lunch 30% GDA	Calories	Sugar	Fat	Saturates	Salt
GDA target	600	27	21	6	1.8

1 *hot meatball wrap (This is an occasional treat – high in salt. Watch your salt intake for rest of day.)

	CALORIES	SUGAR	FAT	SATURATES	SALT
	565	**10.3g**	**25.9g**	**11.6g**	**3.4g**
	28%	11%	37%	58%	57%

1 *Hoisin duck wrap (This is an occasional treat – high in salt. Watch your salt intake for rest of day.)
140g fruit salad
1 30g muesli bar

	CALORIES	SUGAR	FAT	SATURATES	SALT
	584	**34.5g**	**23.0g**	**4.4g**	**2.9g**
	29%	38%	33%	22%	48%

1 *emmental cheese and mushroom panini
1 banana

	CALORIES	SUGAR	FAT	SATURATES	SALT
	549	**22.9g**	**18.5g**	**6.2g**	**1.8g**
	27%	25%	26%	31%	30%

200g *spicy chicken noodle salad (This is an occasional treat – high in salt. Watch your salt intake for rest of day.)
25g dark chocolate

	CALORIES	SUGAR	FAT	SATURATES	SALT
	589	**15.8g**	**26.3g**	**5.8g**	**3.1g**
	29%	18%	38%	29%	52%

1 *egg mayonnaise and mustard cress sandwich (from healthy range)
1 currant bun

	CALORIES	SUGAR	FAT	SATURATES	SALT
	518	**13.4g**	**16.3g**	**1.1g**	**1.7g**
	26%	15%	23%	6%	28%

1 small baked potato with
100g tuna mayonnaise
1 piece of fruit

	CALORIES	SUGAR	FAT	SATURATES	SALT
	572	**16.7g**	**23.5g**	**3.5g**	**0.9g**
	29%	19%	34%	18%	15%

1 bagel topped with
40g light soft cheese and
50g hot-smoked salmon
1 small banana sliced into
1 tbsp natural yogurt and
2 tbsp oats

	CALORIES	SUGAR	FAT	SATURATES	SALT
	577	**27.0g**	**17.6g**	**5.9g**	**2.4g**
	29%	30%	25%	30%	40%

(continued)

Lunch 30% GDA	Calories	Sugar	Fat	Saturates	Salt
GDA target	600	27	21	6	1.8

1 large baked potato *with*
140 g vegetarian chilli
1 sultana scone *with*
2 tsp reduced-fat spread *and*
  2 tsp jam

CALORIES	SUGAR	FAT	SATURATES	SALT
589	23.6g	10.2g	3.2g	1.8g
29%	26%	15%	16%	30%

Ham and cheese sandwich,
  made with:
2 slices wholemeal bread *with*
  2 tsp reduced-fat spread,
1 slice breaded ham,
1 slice cheddar cheese,
1 tsp reduced-fat mayonnaise,
  handful lettuce and 1 sliced
  tomato.
1 large (140 g) fruit salad *with*
3 tbsp natural yogurt

CALORIES	SUGAR	FAT	SATURATES	SALT
532	30.1g	19g	6g	2.0g
27%	33%	27%	30%	33%

Tuna salad:
Large dessert bowl of mixed
  salad
1 tbsp fat-free dressing.
1 can (200 g) tuna in water,
  drained and flaked
1 large wholemeal roll
1 apple
1 teacake *with*
1 tsp reduced-fat spread

CALORIES	SUGAR	FAT	SATURATES	SALT
596	31g	9.5g	2.9g	1.3g
30%	34%	14%	15%	22%

LUNCH PLANNER

Lunch 30% GDA	Calories	Sugar	Fat	Saturates	Salt
GDA target	510	23	18	5.1	1.8

	CALORIES	SUGAR	FAT	SATURATES	SALT
200g baked potato *with* 150g *chilli con carne 1 apple	**501** 29%	**17.4g** 23%	**11.8g** 20%	**4.3g** 25%	**1.2g** 20%
200g baked potato *with* 4tbsp (reduced sugar and salt) baked beans *and* 1tsp grated cheese 140g fruit salad *with* 1tbsp natural yogurt	**506** 30%	**30.9g** 40%	**8.9g** 15%	**5.0g** 29%	**1.5g** 25%
2 slices wholemeal toast *with* 2tsp reduced-fat spread, *topped with* 2 poached eggs 1 small banana *sliced into* 1tbsp natural yogurt *and* 2tbsp oats	**507** 30%	**21.8g** 28%	**19.8g** 33%	**6.2g** 36%	**1.3g** 22%
130–150g pack *sushi 1 toasted teacake *with* 2tsp reduced-fat spread handful of grapes	**490** 29%	**22.3g** 29%	**15.9g** 27%	**4.0g** 24%	**1.9g** 32%
2 slices wholemeal toast *with* 100g sardines canned in tomato sauce 1 slice melon and 2 Scotch pancakes	**510** 30%	**22.5g** 29%	**17.9g** 30%	**3.5g** 21%	**1.8g** 30%
200g *prawn salad *with* large granary roll *and* 140g fruit salad	**505** 30%	**25.3g** 33%	**20.9g** 35%	**1.7g** 10%	**2.1g** 35%
300g *fresh minestrone soup *with* small wholemeal roll *and* 2tsp reduced-fat spread 1 small banana *with* 1tbsp natural yogurt *and* 3tbsp oats	**455** 27%	**29.3g** 38%	**13.6g** 23%	**3.4g** 20%	**2.2g** 37%

(continued)

Lunch 30% GDA	Calories	Sugar	Fat	Saturates	Salt
GDA target	510	23	18	5.1	1.8

1 tortilla wrap *with*
75 g *ready-roasted chicken (without skin) *and* handful shredded lettuce *and*
1 tbsp reduced-fat Caesar dressing
1 tea cake *with* 1 tsp jam

CALORIES	SUGAR	FAT	SATURATES	SALT
508	18.1g	9.9g	4.7g	1.3g
30%	24%	17%	28%	22%

190 g wholemeal pitta bread *filled with* 3 *falafel, 1 tbsp reduced-fat houmous *and* diced red pepper and onion
140 g fruit salad *and* 1 tbsp Fromage frais

CALORIES	SUGAR	FAT	SATURATES	SALT
460	25.0g	14.9g	3.6g	1.8g
27%	33%	25%	21%	30%

250 g *char-grilled vegetable and couscous salad with
1 tbsp reduced-fat *houmous and crudités (choose two from: 1 carrot, 1 yellow pepper, 4 broccoli florets, 2 celery sticks)
1 mini pitta bread

CALORIES	SUGAR	FAT	SATURATES	SALT
510	20.4g	18g	5.1g	1.6g
20%	27%	30%	30%	27%

DINNER PLANNER

Dinner GDA 30%	Calories	Sugar	Fat	Saturates	Salt
GDA target	600	27	21	6	1.8

80 g roast pork with
200 g roast potatoes (4–5 small)
   with gravy and
2 × 80 g portions vegetables

CALORIES	SUGAR	FAT	SATURATES	SALT
565	6.4g	19.2g	3.3g	1.1g
28%	7%	27%	17%	18%

400 g *tomato and mozzarella
   pasta bake with
a large mixed salad and
1 tbsp *fat-free dressing
1 × 25 g pot fruit yogurt

CALORIES	SUGAR	FAT	SATURATES	SALT
597	24.6g	13.5g	5.0g	1.7g
30%	27%	19%	25%	28%

300 g *shepherd's pie with
2 × 80 g portions vegetables
80 g *fruit crumble and
2 tbsp *reduced-fat custard

CALORIES	SUGAR	FAT	SATURATES	SALT
600	40.9g	17.4g	3.6g	2.0g
30%	45%	25%	18%	33%

190 g *individual cheese and
   tomato pizza with extra sliced
   vegetables as a topping (e.g.
   peppers, onion, mushrooms)
   and
a large mixed salad with
1 tbsp fat-free dressing
1 kiwi fruit

CALORIES	SUGAR	FAT	SATURATES	SALT
575	29.4g	14.7g	5.5g	2.5g
29%	33%	21%	28%	42%

400 g *lamb rogan josh with
100 g rice plus
1 mini naan bread

CALORIES	SUGAR	FAT	SATURATES	SALT
593	6.8g	6.7g	2.9g	1.1g
30%	8%	10%	15%	18%

300 g *wild mushroom risotto
2 × 80 g portions vegetables or
large mixed salad
1 small slice sponge cake

CALORIES	SUGAR	FAT	SATURATES	SALT
576	22.2g	24.0g	6.1g	2.9g
29%	25%	34%	31%	48%

Tuna with balsamic onions
See recipe on page 154

CALORIES	SUGAR	FAT	SATURATES	SALT
589	5.5g	20.6g	5.9g	0.7g
29%	6%	29%	30%	12%

1 portion **Lamb Pilau**
See recipe on page 154

CALORIES	SUGAR	FAT	SATURATES	SALT
600	15.8g	20.5g	5.8g	0.6g
30%	18%	29%	29%	10%

(continued)

Dinner GDA 30%	Calories	Sugar	Fat	Saturates	Salt
GDA target	600	27	21	6	1.8

1 portion **Tomato and feta pasta**
See recipe on page 155
Large mixed salad *with*
1 tbsp fat-free dressing

CALORIES	SUGAR	FAT	SATURATES	SALT
550	22.1g	16.6g	6.9g	2.7g
28%	25%	24%	35%	45%

1 portion **Chicken jalfrezi**
See recipe on page 155
(A little high in salt- so have
    occasionally and watch salt
    intake for rest of the day.)

CALORIES	SUGAR	FAT	SATURATES	SALT
592	12.2g	17.7g	1.4g	2.7g
30%	14%	25%	7%	45%

DINNER RECIPES

Tuna with balsamic onions (serves 1)

1 red onion, peeled and sliced
3 tsp olive oil
130 ml balsamic vinegar
4 medium potatoes, peeled and sliced
160 g tuna steak
Juice 1 lemon
Ground black pepper for seasoning
Large handful rocket leaves
25 g goat's cheese, crumbled

1 In a saucepan, soften the onion in 1 tsp olive oil for about 5 minutes.

2 Add the balsamic vinegar and cook over a gentle heat until reduced and syrupy (about 10–15 minutes).

3 Boil the potato slices in water for 7–8 minutes until tender, drain and set aside.

4 Brush 1 tsp olive oil over the tuna steak, season with black pepper and grill or griddle for 2–3 minutes on each side.

5 Squeeze the lemon juice over the tuna at the end of cooking.

6 Combine the sliced potatoes, a large handful of rocket and the goat's cheese. Drizzle over 1 tsp olive oil.

7 Place the tuna steak on the leaves and top the tuna with the onions.

Lamb pilau (serves 4)

2 tbsp pine nuts
1 tsp sunflower oil
1 red onion, peeled and sliced
2 cinnamon sticks
500 g lean lamb neck fillet, cubed
250 g basmati rice (dry weight)
500 ml low-salt stock made from concentrate or cube
12 soft dried apricots, diced
2 tbsp fresh mint, chopped

1 Dry fry the pine nuts until lightly browned. Set aside.

2 In another frying pan, soften the onion in the oil and add the cinnamon sticks.

3 Turn up the heat and add the cubed lamb. Brown the meat and then tip in the basmati rice and cook for 1 minute, stirring all the time.

4 Pour in the stock and add the dried apricots.

5 Reduce the heat, cover and simmer for 20–25 minutes until all the stock has been absorbed. Check the rice is cooked through.

6 Sprinkle in the pine nuts and mint and serve.

Tomato and feta pasta
(serves 4)

300 g pasta (dry weight)
2 tsp sunflower oil
1 onion, peeled and sliced
1 clove garlic, peeled and crushed
2 × 400 g cans chopped tomatoes
Ground black pepper for seasoning
1 tsp dried oregano or basil
2 tbsp fresh parsley, chopped
175 g feta cheese, cubed

1 Cook the pasta according to the packet instructions.

2 In a frying pan, soften the onion and crushed garlic in the oil. Stir in the chopped tomatoes. Season with black pepper and oregano or basil, bring to the boil and simmer, uncovered, for 10 minutes.

3 Drain the pasta and combine with the tomato sauce.

4 Stir in the parsley and feta cheese and serve.

Chicken jalfrezi
(serves 4)

400 g chicken breast, skinless and boneless, cubed
2 tsp sunflower oil
150 g mushrooms, sliced
2 onions, peeled and sliced
2 green peppers, deseeded and sliced into strips
500 g jalfrezi sauce
300 g basmati rice (dry weight)

1 Stir fry the chicken breast in the oil until lightly browned and add the mushrooms, onions and peppers. Cook until they soften, about 10 minutes.

2 Add the jalfrezi sauce and heat through until bubbling and the chicken is cooked.

3 Cook the rice according to the packet instructions.

4 Serve the curry sauce on top of the rice.

DINNER PLANNER

Dinners (30% GDA)	Calories	Sugar	Fat	Saturates	Salt
GDA target	510	23	18	5.1	1.8
300 g *shepherd's pie with 2 × 80 g portions vegetables 200 g canned *reduced-fat rice pudding with 1 tsp jam	452 27%	27.7g 36%	8.3g 14%	4.3g 25%	1.8g 30%
225 g *liver and onions with 3 medium potatoes, mashed and 2 × 80 g portions vegetables	505 30%	12.4g 16%	18g 30%	5.0g 29%	1.8g 30%
450 g Lancashire hotpot with 2 × 80 g portions vegetables	510 30%	11.8g 15%	22.6g 38%	11.0g 65%	2.4g 40%
300 g *tomato and cheese spaghetti with a large mixed salad and 1 tbsp *fat-free dressing 1 pot fruit yogurt 1 apple	491 29%	24.0g 31%	14.3g 24%	4.3g 25%	2.3g 38%
150 g *four-cheese pizza with a large green salad and 1 tbsp *fat-free dressing 100 g fruit salad	510 30%	21.1g 28%	17.0g 28%	6.8g 40%	1.9g 32%
Chinese spiced tofu *See recipe on page 157* 1 small banana	510 30%	20.8g 27%	19.7g 33%	3.4g 20%	2.1g 35%
Bulgur wheat and squash salad *See recipe on page 157*	510 30%	15.6g 20%	13.3g 22%	6.6g 39%	1.5g 25%
Sticky chicken *See recipe on page 157*	495 29%	12.4g 16%	15.2g 25%	3.4g 20%	0.8g 13%
Turkey Bolognese *See recipe on page 158*	510 30%	12.0g 16%	13.2g 22%	2.7g 16%	1.6g 27%
Salmon and couscous surprise *See recipe on page 158*	508 30%	13.7g 18%	21.0g 35%	3.6g 21%	0.7g 12%

RECIPES

All recipes serve 1, but can be doubled or tripled for more people.

Chinese spiced tofu

125 g tofu
1 tsp sunflower oil
200 g pack prepared stir fry
  vegetables
60 g noodles (dry weight)
2 tsp sesame oil
1 tsp Chinese five-spice powder
2 tsp soy sauce

1 In a large pan or wok, brown the tofu in the oil.

2 Remove the tofu from the pan to a plate with a slotted spoon and keep warm. Quickly stir fry the selection of vegetables in the same oil.

3 In a large pan of water, cook the noodles according to the packet instructions.

4 Meanwhile, combine the sesame oil, Chinese five-spice powder and soy sauce in a bowl. Return the tofu to the stir-fried vegetables, add the sesame/soy mixture and stir well. Bring quickly to the boil and serve with drained noodles.

Bulgur wheat and squash salad

75 g bulgur wheat (dry weight)
250 g butternut squash, peeled and
  sliced
Spray oil
50 g feta cheese, cubed
Handful fresh sage, chopped, or
  1 tsp dried sage
Ground black pepper for seasoning
Juice ½ lemon
1 tsp clear honey

1 Cook the bulgur wheat according to the packet instructions.

2 Place the prepared squash in a roasting tin and spray lightly with the oil. Roast in a pre-heated oven at Gas Mark 4, 180 °C until starting to soften.

3 Combine the cooked bulgur wheat, roasted squash and feta cheese.

4 Add some the chopped sage leaves and season with black pepper.

5 Combine the lemon juice and honey and drizzle over the salad.

Sticky chicken

Juice 1 lemon
2 tsp clear honey
1 tsp olive oil
3 chicken drumsticks or chicken
   thighs, skin on
2 small potatoes, peeled and
   quartered
2–3 slices lemon
1–2 sprigs fresh rosemary and
   thyme
2 × 80 g portions vegetables

1 Combine the lemon juice with the honey and olive oil.

2 Arrange chicken pieces in small roasting tray with potatoes.

3 Tuck in the lemon wedges and herbs and drizzle over the lemon and honey mixture.

4 Roast for 35–40 mins in a pre-heated oven at Gas Mark 4, 180 °C.

5 Serve immediately with 2 × 80 g portions of vegetables.

Turkey bolognese

110 g turkey mince
½ onion, peeled and diced
Handful mushrooms, sliced
150 g bolognese sauce
80 g spaghetti or pasta shapes (dry
   weight)

1 Dry fry the mince in a non-stick pan, stirring all the time until beginning to brown.

2 Add the onion and mushrooms and continue to stir. Cook for 6–7 minutes until softened.

3 Add bolognese sauce and simmer for 10 minutes.

4 Cook the pasta according to packet instructions.

5 Serve the cooked sauce on a bed of drained pasta.

Salmon and couscous surprise

75 g couscous (dry weight)
Juice 1 lemon
2 tsp dried dill
2 spring onions, sliced
2 sun-dried tomatoes, sliced
100 g salmon fillet
2 × 80 g portions vegetables

1 Cook the couscous according to the packet instructions, adding ¾ of the lemon juice and 1 tsp dried dill.

2 Pile the cooked couscous in the centre of a large sheet of tin foil.

3 Top with the onion and tomato, followed by the salmon fillet. Drizzle over the remaining lemon juice and dill.

4 Scrunch up the foil to form a sealed pouch and place on a baking sheet.

5 Bake for 20–25 minutes in a pre-heated oven at Gas Mark 4, 170 °C.

6 Serve in the foil with 2 × 80 g portions of vegetables.

SNACK PLANNER

Snack 10% GDA	Calories	Sugar	Fat	Saturates	Salt
GDA target	200	9	7	2	0.6
40 g fruit n' fibre cereal *with* 140 ml semi-skimmed milk	**200** 10%	**15.7g** 17%	**4.2g** 6%	**2.5g** 13%	**0.5g** 8%
2 slices *melba toast with* 30 g *mushroom pâté*	**200** 10%	**1.3g** 1%	**5.2g** 7%	**1.9g** 10%	**0.3g** 5%
half a 30 g packet or 15 g packet mini rice cakes a large handful grapes and 1 kiwi fruit	**182** 91%	**15g** 17%	**2.7g** 4%	**0.4g** 2%	**1.5g** 25%
1 fruited and spiced toasted English muffin *with* 1 tsp reduced-fat spread	**200** 10%	**9.1g** 10%	**6.7g** 10%	**2.3g** 12%	**0.6g** 10%
40 g dark chocolate	**196** 10%	**20.4g** 23%	**12.2g** 17%	**7.4g** 37%	**0.05g** 1%
2 wheat biscuits 125 ml semi-skimmed milk 1 tsp mixed nuts	**200** 10%	**6.6g** 7%	**6.1g** 9%	**2.0g** 10%	**0.4g** 7%
2 × 1 cm (½ in) slices malt loaf	**185** 9%	**16.8g** 19%	**1.3g** 2%	**0.9g** 5%	**0.3g** 5%
1 toasted currant bun *with* 1 slice pineapple	**200** 10%	**16.8g** 19%	**3.5g** 5%	**1.1g** 6%	**0.4g** 7%
3 water biscuits *topped with* 25 g blue stilton and a small handful grapes	**200** 10%	**6.2g** 7%	**9.4g** 13%	**7.4g** 37%	**0.8g** 14%
1 (27 g) sachet instant plain porridge made up according to packet instructions made with skimmed milk. Stir in 2 chopped, dried apricots	**200** 10%	**13.9g** 15%	**5.5g** 8%	**2.3g** 12%	**0.2g** 3%

SNACK PLANNER

Snack 10% GDA	Calories	Sugar	Fat	Saturates	Salt
GDA target	170	7.6	6.0	1.7	0.6
30 g bran flakes *with* 125 ml semi-skimmed milk	CALORIES 153 10%	SUGAR 10.7g 14%	FAT 2.8g 5%	SATURATES 1.4g 8%	SALT 0.5g 8%
2 oatcakes *with* 1 tbsp cottage cheese	CALORIES 139 8%	SUGAR 1.9g 2%	FAT 5.2g 9%	SATURATES 2.1g 12%	SALT 1.0g 17%
3 rice cakes *topped with* 1½ tbsp reduced-fat *houmous	CALORIES 147 9%	SUGAR 1.1g 1%	FAT 5.9g 10%	SATURATES 1.0g 6%	SALT 0.7g 12%
2 satsumas, 1 toasted crumpet *with* 1 tsp reduced-fat spread	CALORIES 122 7%	SUGAR 8.6g 11%	FAT 2.8g 5%	SATURATES 1.0g 6%	SALT 0.6g 10%
20 g milk chocolate-coated peanuts	CALORIES 109 6%	SUGAR 5.8g 8%	FAT 7.1g 12%	SATURATES 2.8g 16%	SALT 0.05g 1%
1 slice malt loaf and a large handful of grapes	CALORIES 134 8%	SUGAR 15.7g 21%	FAT 0.7g 1%	SATURATES 0.4g 2%	SALT 0.1g 2%
1 currant bun	CALORIES 168 10%	SUGAR 9.1g 12%	FAT 3.4g 6%	SATURATES 1.1g 6%	SALT 0.4g 6%
3 water biscuits *with* 1 tsp extra light soft cheese and 1 slice wafer thin ham 1 apple	CALORIES 161 9%	SUGAR 12.2g 16%	FAT 3.1g 5%	SATURATES 1.7g 10%	SALT 1.0g 17%
27 g sachet instant plain porridge made up according to packet instructions	CALORIES 170 10%	SUGAR 8.7g 11%	FAT 5.4g 9%	SATURATES 2.3g 14%	SALT 0.2g 3%

YOUR OWN GDA FOOD LIST

As you get more and more familiar with GDAs, you will start to find your own favourite meals and snacks. To save yourself time in the future, it will be useful for you to add them into the table below.

GDA FOOD LIST

Meal or snack	Calories	Sugar	Fat	Saturates	Salt

9 THE GDA DIET TOP TIPS

Cooking from scratch can mean it's more difficult to keep track of your GDAs, so I have put together some of my favourite healthy cooking tips, a comprehensive portion guide and a guide to all the 'extras' like soft drinks and alcohol – to ensure that whatever you're eating or drinking you can choose to keep on the right side of your GDAs.

TIPS FOR SHOPPING ON A BUDGET

We all have to look after the pennies a little more carefully these days, but that doesn't have to be at the expense of your health or your waistline. Economical food and money-saving menu planning can be bursting with good nutrition and as my 7-day plans for people on a budget show (see pages 104 and 134), they can also be perfect for weight control. Whether or not you are following the budget plans, the next few pages offer something for anyone who doesn't like wasting money.

Recent research has shown that each of us throw away approximately £600-worth of food each year. Just imagine what you could do with that money. Go on holiday? Buy new clothes? A new sofa? Bill payments? So here are my top tips for keeping an eye on the pennies:

▶ Keep your fresh fruit and vegetables in the chill compartment of the fridge so that they last longer.
▶ Think about portion sizes when serving up meals. Are you continually scraping food into the bin? Try not to prepare

more food than you need. For example, a single mugful of dry, uncooked rice will serve four adults. So if you're feeding two children and two adults, you're likely to need only two-thirds of a mugful.

▶ Use up leftovers and *think* before you throw food away. Even the most basic of foods can be brought back to life in soups, casseroles, sauces or stock. With a little imagination you can rustle up all sorts of exciting new meals from family leftovers.

Don't be tempted to 'eat up' just to prevent wastage. Rather than risk progress on your diet, simply decide to plan more effectively next time.

▶ If you've got whole portions of meals left over, put them in the freezer for another day when you're short of time.

▶ If you focus on managing your food budget more effectively, you will find it easier to stay on your diet plan and cut back your portion sizes too.

Better food management

▶ **Use your freezer.** It's useful to keep a good stock of healthy freezer food for those days when you've run out of fresh vegetables. Use your freezer to benefit from supermarket special offers to cut costs but keep an eye on the 'use by' dates.

▶ **Know your use-by and sell-by dates.** Stick to the dates printed on packaging, and if something is likely to reach its use-by date before you have a chance to consume it, don't buy it. Food might last a little longer if you freeze it, but you should always follow food labelling instructions carefully to avoid health risks. Get into the habit of checking dates regularly so you know what to eat up and when.

▶ **Storing fruit and vegetables.** Most food wastage advice applies to this food group, but by buying unbruised and fresh produce and storing it correctly you can keep it for longer and avoid tipping your money into the bin.

▶ **Divide large packets of food** (especially chicken and fish) into smaller portions and store them in the freezer or fridge in separate containers. Splitting the pack means you'll only have to defrost the required amounts at any one time so the other portions will last a lot longer. (It also means you won't prepare – and eat – more than you need.)

▶ **If you don't buy it you can't eat it.** Remember to buy everything you need for your diet in advance – and never shop for food when you're hungry, as you're more likely to make bad choices. Help yourself, by planning ahead, to make sure that high-fat and sugary foods don't make it into your basket.

Store-cupboard essentials

▶ **Tinned and packet foods.** Keep a good selection of the staple foods that your family love, such as baked beans, dried fruit, pasta and rice. Most of these ingredients have a long shelf life, which means you can rely on them as stand-bys to create quick, delicious meals, or use them as a basis to mix in leftovers. Replace them once they've gone to ensure the cupboard remains fully stocked. (It's useful to keep a list on the inside of the cupboard as a reminder.)

▶ **Your daily loaf.** Bread is one of the biggest victims of food waste. We throw away millions of slices in the UK every day. To keep your loaf alive, freeze it and take slices out of the freezer when you want to toast it. Split big loaves in half and thaw them when needed, depending on how soon you're likely to eat it.

► **Buy in season.** Seasonal food usually costs less, especially if it is grown naturally, in local farms. Seasonal food also tastes better, and if you buy produce that is locally grown not only is it likely to be more fresh, it won't have run up air-miles, meaning it's good for the environment too.

► **Shop late.** Supermarkets often make price cuts at the end of the working day. Take a trip to a store at around 8 pm and you're very likely to find some good bargains with price cuts of 50% or more, which you can either eat quickly or freeze to extend its shelf life.

► **Buy loose fresh fruit and vegetables.** Picking and packing loose fruit and vegetables instead of choosing pre-packed bags can give you precious savings over time. Root vegetables are often better value per kilogram when bought loose. You're also more likely to buy only the amount you need, so there's less wastage. Large bags of fruit and vegetables that have been discounted are only good value if you're definitely going to use them all before they go off.

► **Buy own brands and value ranges.** Don't be fooled into thinking that premium brands are always better for you. Premium brands may contain higher levels of fat, salt or sugar. Try some of your supermarket's own brands and also give the 'basic' or 'value' range a go. I bet you won't notice any difference in taste. Use the GDA labels to see for yourself that they're just as good for you as the posh nosh.

In the 'at a glance' meal plan tables for the 7-day plan on a budget, you can see all the budget ranges I have used. (See pages 212–223)

► **Buy online.** If you use online shopping facilities you're more likely to stick to your shopping list rather than getting sucked into buying special offers that you're never going to eat, or buying tempting treats that you know you shouldn't eat.

SAVVY GDA-SAVING TIPS

The GDA 7-day eating plans are packed full of convenience meals and snacks to help you see how easy it is to follow the GDA Diet without having to spend hours in the kitchen preparing special meals. If, like me, you cook some meals from scratch and use some ready-meals during an average week – that's OK. If you decide you want to make some of your meals from scratch, go right ahead and do that too, but please read my tips (following) on how to keep your home-cooked dishes GDA-friendly.

There are also plenty of extra 'hidden calories' in the fats and sugars in many sauces and dressings, drinks and snacks that can send your overall GDAs for the day soaring. These can all be avoided with just a little bit of know-how.

Portion sizes

Portion sizes cause a lot of confusion and it's very easy to get used to eating far more than we need. It is a common route to weight gain. My average portion guide to every day staple foods will help you take a look at your normal portion sizes and see if you think you can cut down.

Sauces and Gravies

White sauce, traditionally called béchamel sauce is made by making a roux (of melted butter and flour) blended with milk. A basic white sauce can then be flavoured by adding cheese, onion, mustard, parsley or other herbs and vegetables. A typical serving of 100 g of béchamel sauce can contain 170 calories (8.5% GDA) and 9.5 g fat (13.5% GDA).

My low-fat alternative white sauce can be flavoured in exactly the same way as a traditional béchamel. A 100 g serving will provide just 40 calories (2% GDA) and 0.1 g fat (7% GDA).

Low fat white sauce (2 servings)

200 ml skimmed milk
2-3 tsp cornflour

1 Make a paste with the cornflour and a little water

2 Add the milk to the cornflour paste

3 Gently heat, stirring all the time

4 As the milk thickens, slowly bring to simmering point for 2-3 minutes

5 If the sauce needs more thickening, remove from the heat and add a little more cornflour paste

6 Return to the heat and bring to simmering point as before

7 Add any cheese, or flavourings before serving (see special note for onion sauce 168)

GDA Information per 100 ml serving:

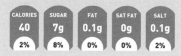

CALORIES	SUGAR	FAT	SAT FAT	SALT
40	7g	0.1g	0g	0.1g
2%	8%	0%	0%	2%

White sauce adaptations (2 servings)

Cheese sauce

Add 50 g grated mature cheddar cheese and 1 tsp English mustard

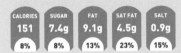

CALORIES	SUGAR	FAT	SAT FAT	SALT
151	7.4g	9.1g	4.5g	0.9g
8%	8%	13%	23%	15%

Parsley sauce

Add 2 tablespoons of finely chopped fresh parsley or 3 teaspoons of dried chopped parsley

GDA information – as plain white sauce

Onion sauce

1 onion, peeled and finely chopped or grated. Add the onion at to the milk at the beginning before you start heating the milk

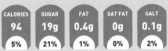

CALORIES	SUGAR	FAT	SAT FAT	SALT
94	19g	0.4g	0g	0.1g
5%	21%	1%	0%	2%

Mustard sauce

Add 3 tsp wholegrain mustard.

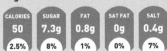

CALORIES	SUGAR	FAT	SAT FAT	SALT
50	7.3g	0.8g	0g	0.4g
2.5%	8%	1%	0%	7%

Low fat/low salt gravy (2 servings)

250 ml Meat juices from roasting joint
Ice cubes
2–3 teaspoons cornflour or plain flour
Extra water if needed

1 Drain the meat juices from the roasting tin in the normal way into a clear measuring jug or glass bowl.

2 Add a large handful of ice cubes and place the juices in the fridge or freezer if in a hurry

3 After 10–15 minutes remove the chilled meat juices from the fridge. The fat will have solidified and will be a creamy white colour so easily visible.

4 Skim the fat from the juices with a spoon and add them back to the meat roasting tray.

5 Mix the flour with a little water into a paste and add to the juices

6 Over a gentle heat, stir continuously until the gravy thickens

7 Serve immediately

GDA information per 120ml serving:

CALORIES	SUGAR	FAT	SAT FAT	SALT
35	2g	2g	1g	0.4g
1.7%	2%	3%	10%	7%

Salads and dressings

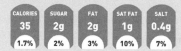

Low fat herby vinaigrette

Makes enough dressing to serve 2 large servings of salad
3 tbsp very low fat French dressing
3 tbsp fresh tarragon, chopped- could also use basil, sage or parsley
1/4 tsp grain mustard salt and pepper

GDA information per serving:

CALORIES	SUGAR	FAT	SAT FAT	SALT
39	4g	3g	0.5g	0.4g
2%	4%	4%	1%	7%

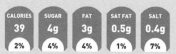

Very low fat mayonnaise

Perfect to dress salads or for home made low fat coleslaw and potato salad
2 tablespoons very low fat mayonnaise
2 tablespoons low fat natural yoghurt
Herbs and spices of choice (optional)

1 Blend all the ingredients together until well combined.

2 Add herbs (e.g. basil), spices (e.g. curry powder) or crushed garlic, for extra flavour.

GDA information per 15g serving:

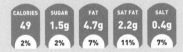

CALORIES	SUGAR	FAT	SAT FAT	SALT
49	1.5g	4.7g	2.2g	0.4g
2%	2%	7%	11%	7%

Basic tomato sauce for pasta (4 servings)

1 tsp sunflower oil
2 cloves garlic, crushed
1 medium onion, finely chopped
1 × 400g can chopped tomatoes, undrained
2 tbsp balsamic vinegar
2 teaspoons tomato puree
2 teaspoons dried mixed herbs
Freshly ground black pepper

1 Heat oil in a large pan.

2 Sauté garlic and onions on low heat until softened, about 5 minutes.

3 Add tomatoes, balsamic vinegar and tomato paste. Bring to a boil, then reduce to a simmer.

4 Add herbs and simmer uncovered for 15 minutes.

GDA information per serving:

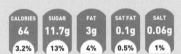

CALORIES	SUGAR	FAT	SAT FAT	SALT
64	11.7g	3g	0.1g	0.06g
3.2%	13%	4%	0.5%	1%

Variations:
You can add fish, prawns, chopped vegetables, smokey bacon to this sauce or use it as a base to make your own bolognaise. Though these will increase the calorie content.

OTHER USEFUL TIPS TO SAVE CALORIES, FATS, SUGARS AND SALT

Cooking methods

Dry frying: You don't have to add extra oil or fat to the pan when cooking. Meat can be dry fried for casseroles, pasta dishes and stews. Choose lean cuts of meat and place in a cold frying pan. Place the plan over a medium heat and even the leanest meat will still contain enough fat to stop the meat from sticking to the pan.

Steaming and microwaving: These methods help vegetables to retain vitamins and minerals.

Boiling: If you prefer to boil your vegetables try to use the minimum water possible and cook as quickly as possible by adding the vegetables to the water when it is boiling.

Mashed potato

Instead of adding butter and milk to mashed potato in the traditional way, try using a dash of semi-skimmed milk and whisk the potatoes with an electric whisk. They'll be creamy and light but with fewer calories and less fat than the full fat version.

Likely savings: 90 calories (4.5%) 10 g fat (14%) in a typical serving.

Roast potatoes

If you can't imagine a Sunday roast without roasties, try dry roasting. Part-boil the potatoes for 10 minutes, drain and shake them in the saucepan with the lid on, to make them fluffy. Then use spray oil to give them a very light coating and roast in a hot oven for around 30 minutes or until golden brown.

Likely savings: up to 180 calories (9%) and 20 g fat (29%) in a typical serving.

Chips

Make potato wedges instead of home-made chips. Cut potatoes into thick wedges (leave the skins on). There's no need to part-boil; just place them in a roasting tin and spray with oil. Cook in a hot oven for 30-40 minutes.

Likely savings: 260 kals (13% GDA) 20 g fat (29% GDA).

Sandwiches

Use medium-sliced bread for sandwiches and it's fine to use a mixture of different breads – such as white, wholemeal and granary. If you need to use a spread then choose a low-fat variety and try to stick to around 1 tsp or 7 g of spread per slice of bread.

Alternatives to spreads: If you are using a 'wet' filling, such as tuna with low fat mayonnaise, then you probably don't need to use spread. Pickles also keep sandwiches moist (but keep an eye on the GDA label because some pickles can very salty). Sliced tomatoes, beetroot and salad leaves work too; they are low-calorie and GDA-friendly .

Custard and sweet sauces

There are some great reduced-fat and low-sugar 'ready made' custards available, but if you prefer to make your own, then try using an artificial sweetener and skimmed or semi-skimmed milk.

Tea and coffee

There is no reason to avoid tea and coffee when you are trying to lose weight and if you take your cuppa with milk, the amount of milk most of us use is negligible so don't worry about that too much. The thing to be wary of taking sugar in your brew.

Each teaspoon of sugar provides 5 g (6% GDA) of your GDA for sugars. If you have 3 sugars per cup, and have 6 cups a day that means you'll have used up all 100% of your

GDA for sugar just on your drinks. There are some very good artificial sweeteners available which don't have the unpleasant aftertaste you might remember from a few years ago. Switching to a sweetener or giving up sugar in hot drinks can be a major way to reduce sugar and calorie intake for some people, so don't under estimate the difference it could make. An average of 3–4 cups of tea or coffee without sugar a day is fine and counts towards your body's daily need for fluids.

Be careful: if you stop at the coffee shop to pick up a latte or cappuccino don't forget to add it to your GDAs.

Grande latte (regular milk)

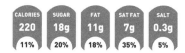

CALORIES	SUGAR	FAT	SAT FAT	SALT
220	18g	11g	7g	0.3g
11%	20%	18%	35%	5%

Grande latte (skinny)

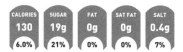

CALORIES	SUGAR	FAT	SAT FAT	SALT
130	19g	0g	0g	0.4g
6.0%	21%	0%	0%	7%

Other soft drinks

A typical can of full-sugar fizzy drink contains 35 g sugar (38% GDA) so it's easy to see how soft drinks can make a significant contribution to your daily calorie intake. If you enjoy fizzy drinks then swapping to a diet variety will instantly save all of that sugar and all of those calories. Similarly, swapping from full-sugar squash drinks to no-added-sugar or diet varieties can make huge savings.

Looking at the GDA labels of soft drinks is a fantastic way to learn how to CHECK, COMPARE and CHOOSE.

Alcohol

Alcohol contains what nutritionists call 'empty calories'. These are calories that have absolutely no nutritional value: no vitamins, minerals, fibre or protein. Alcohol contains 7 calories per gram, which puts it second only to fat, at 9 calories per gram, in high calorific value.

Let's imagine you have two large glasses of wine each evening. That's 330 empty calories each night; or 2310 empty calories in one week. Remember that your total GDA for calories is 2000 per day (or 1700 per day on the GDA lower-calorie plan). That means you would be drinking more than one-day's worth of calories per week in booze alone. If you enjoy the occasional drink then there is no need to give up alcohol altogether, but if you are trying to lose weight you must be aware of the contribution your alcohol intake has on your total calorie intake.

The table below shows the calorie values and %GDA for a selection of popular drinks at standard pub measures:

Alcoholic drink	Calories	% GDA
Large glass dry white wine (2 units)	CALORIES 165	8%
½ pint regular strength lager (1 units)	CALORIES 65	3%
Gin and tonic (1 units)	CALORIES 114	6%
Vodka and orange juice (1 units)	CALORIES 164	8%

(continued)

Alcoholic drink	Calories	% GDA
Southern Comfort and lemonade (1 units)	**193** / 10%	
Tia Maria and coke (1 units)	**180** / 9%	
Medium glass of red wine (1½ units)	**119** / 6%	
½ pint of cider (1 units)	**103** / 5%	
Glass of champagne (1 units)	**95** / 5%	

The recommended levels for the safe intake of alcohol per week is 14 units for women, and 21 units for men. However, it will be difficult to lose weight if you are consuming these amounts so plan to stay well inside the safe limits. It's recommended that you have at least two or three alcohol-free days each week.

These tips can help you reduce the amount you drink and the calories you consume through alcohol:

► If you drink wine, try changing to wine spritzers, made with half wine and half soda water or sparkling mineral water
► Use diet mixers with spirits
► Choose lager or bitter shandy made with diet lemonade instead regular beer
► Alternate an alcoholic drink with a diet soft drink or sparkling mineral water
► Offer to drive to the pub so you can't drink!

FRUITS, VEGETABLES AND SALADS

Enjoy a wide variety of fruit and vegetable types every day. Aim for five servings daily and choose a mixture of colours to ensure a good mix of nutrients. All fruit and vegetables, including fresh, frozen, canned, dried and pure juices, count towards the five daily servings.

But bear in mind that dried fruit won't fill you up as much as a whole piece of fruit – for 100 calories you can eat an apple, a satsuma and seven strawberries (with a total weight of 250 g) or around 1 tbsp of raisins (with a weight of just 30 g)! You can also count just one small glass of fruit juice towards your five a day.

Salads

When making salads, use a mixture of different leaves; there is a wide variety of mixed leaf salads leaves in all supermarkets (one bag of leaves should serve 2–3 people). Add extra chopped vegetables, such as raw peppers, cucumber, grated carrot, beetroot, tomatoes, onions, watercress, mustard and cress, sliced mushrooms, celery and sweetcorn. Make your salads colourful, with lots of different textures to give you a crunchy, crispy refreshing side-dish or meal. A side-salad should fill a dessert bowl and a main-course salad should fill a dinner plate.

Veggies

When you serve up meals, put the vegetables or salad on the plate first and aim to fill half the plate. This way you are more likely to give yourself smaller portions of the more calorific protein (meat, fish, poultry) and carbohydrate (potatoes, rice, pasta or bread) parts of the meal. If you are using the dressing I have suggested above, your salads and vegetables will be low in calories, fat, saturates, sugar and salt.

One portion of fruit or veg is equivalent to 80 g. Below are some examples of what counts as one portion:

- ▶ 1 apple, banana, pear, orange, or other similar sized fruit
- ▶ 2 plums, satsumas, kiwi fruit, or other similar sized fruit
- ▶ 1/2 a grapefruit or avocado
- ▶ 1 large slice of melon or fresh pineapple
- ▶ 3 heaped tablespoons of vegetables, beans or pulses
- ▶ 3 heaped tablespoons of fruit salad or stewed fruit
- ▶ 1 heaped tablespoon of raisins or sultanas
- ▶ 3 dried apricots
- ▶ 1 cupful of grapes, cherries or berries
- ▶ 1 dessert bowl of salad
- ▶ 1 small glass (150ml) of pure fruit juice

AVERAGE PORTION SIZES FOR STAPLE INGREDIENTS

These average portion sizes are included to help you assess the portion sizes you would normally serve up for yourself and see what you could make smaller. I don't expect you to weigh your food every day, that would be ridiculous, but it might be helpful to know what 120 g of French bread, 120 g white fish or a medium bowl of cereal looks like, so that you can make sure you are eating the right amount for you.

If you start a meal with the right portion size on your plate you will feel full and will be less likely to go back for more. However, if you start your meal with twice the average portion served on your plate, you are very likely to finish it all!

All measurements are for medium servings.

Bread

Medium slice	35 g
Bagel	70 g

Pitta bread	95 g
Chapati	55 g
Crumpet	40 g
French bread 7.5 cm (6 in) slice	100 g
Naan bread	160 g
Fruit bread	35 g
Malt loaf	35 g

Breakfast cereal

All bran	40 g
Corn flakes	30 g
Fruit and fibre	40 g
Muesli	50 g
Rice Krispies	30 g
1 wheat biscuit	20 g

Cheese and cheese dishes

Cheddar	40 g
Cheese quiche	120 g
Cream cheese	30 g
Brie	40 g
Cottage cheese	40 g

Eggs and egg dishes

Boiled egg	57 g
2-egg omelette	120 g
Scrambled egg	60 g
Fried egg	60 g

Fats and oils

I slice bread and butter or hard margarine	10 g
I slice bread and spreadable butter or margarine	7 g

Thin scraping on cracker	2 g
1 tbsp oil	11 g
1 tsp oil	3 g

Fish

White fish	120 g
Oily fish	170 g

Meat and meat dishes

1 rasher lean, back bacon	40 g
Beefburger	60–90 g
Meat casserole/curry	260 g
Mince dish (bolognaise style)	140 g
Meat or chicken pie	120 g
Roast meat	90 g
Steaks off the bone	100 g
Steaks on the bone	166 g
Chicken breast portion (boneless)	130 g
Chicken drumstick (with bone)	165 g
Chicken leg (with bone)	165 g
Ham/chicken/turkey cold slice	25 g
Pork chop (on bone)	165 g
Lasagne	290 g
1 sausage	50 g

Pasta, rice, grains and potatoes

Couscous (1 tbsp)	33 g
Noodles (1 pack, instant)	280 g
Oats (1 tbsp, dry weight)	15 g
Pasta (cooked)	230 g
Rice (cooked)	180 g
Spaghetti (cooked)	220 g
Potatoes	
Baked (with skin)	180 g
Boiled	175 g

Chips	165 g
Mashed (3 tbsp)	180 g
Roast	200 g

Yoghurts and desserts

Individual yoghurt	125 g
Milk pudding	200 g
Fruit pie	110 g
Fruit fool	120 g
Mousse	60 g
Pavlova	100 g
Trifle	170 g
Custard	120 g
Ice cream (soft scoop)	75 g
Sorbet	95 g

Sauces pickles and soups

Hot savoury sauce (cheese, onion etc)	65 g
1 tsp chutney or pickle	10 g
1 tbsp chutney or pickle	33 g
Mayonnaise (with salad)	30 g
Gravy	50 g
Soup	220 g

10 MOVING ON UP

I've shown you how to use the GDA plans and how to pick the right plan for you. We've also looked at simple ways to include more of the nutritional goodies in your diet and keep tabs on the nutrients you need to eat less of.

So what else do you need to make your GDA Diet and lifestyle complete? You've got it ... some activity.

Don't panic! This is going to be easy, and although it may take a little effort to start with I guarantee that after a couple of weeks, being more active will soon become just another enjoyable part of your day-to-day life.

Being active is a really important part of your success and will help you stay in control of your weight and your health for a lifetime. Remember the old-fashioned set of grocer's scales I used to explain energy balance? (See page 182) Now imagine putting the things you eat on one side of the scales and the things you do to burn energy on the other side. How balanced is your lifestyle?

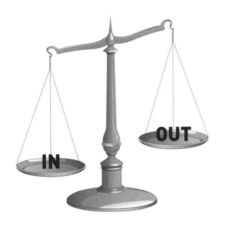

More energy in than going out = Weight gain

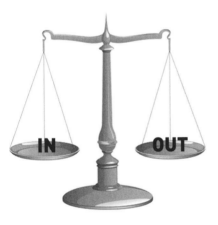

Equal amounts of energy in and energy out = weight maintenance

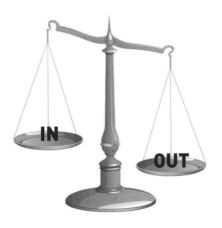

More energy out than going in = weight loss

Of course, there are several ways to shift the balance in favour of weight loss:

▶ You can put all your energy into exercising, so you can get away with eating anything you like without gaining weight. (I could never love exercise this much, so I'd say no thanks!)
▶ You can restrict your eating to such an extent that you make all the calorie savings you need to lose weight without lifting a finger. (I love eating too much to do that.)
▶ **Or you can take an altogether more reasonable approach and choose to save a few calories here and burn a few off there. (Now that sounds more like it!)**

'Nigel has got it so right. Focusing on being active is the best way to keep healthy and stay in shape. So many of my clients come to me thinking I am going to work them into the ground. They are so surprised when we start by looking at their day-to-day activity levels, but they love the results they get!'
Paul Connolly, health and fitness expert

Although I'm no sports fan, I do know that if I don't take regular physical exercise I will have to watch what I eat like a hawk or the pounds start to creep on. Making simple changes to fit activity into your everyday routine does take a bit of getting used to, I admit. But after a couple of weeks it will feel like the norm, believe me – and you'll wonder why you found it so hard before.

Being active is so normal to me these days that I miss it if I don't do something every day. For me the bonus is that I never have to set foot in a gym to keep fit. But of course, if you enjoy a workout don't let me stop you. Just make sure your gym sessions are a bonus on top of your daily activity routine.

In my own case, because I'm maintaining my weight loss rather than trying to lose weight, I know that walking for half an hour or so means I can afford to have a glass of wine occasionally, or the dessert I'd otherwise have to think twice about. If I notice after a holiday or Christmas that my waistband is beginning to pinch, I just step up the walking and cut down on the wine and the puddings, and I'm back to my happy weight again in no time.

If the benefits of daily activity over one or two weekly gym workouts sound too good to be true, here's a challenge for you so you can see for yourself. Start taking a brisk 30-minute walk, or some other activity, every day for two weeks. I'll guarantee that it will help you look and feel much more like you really want to look and feel. Will you take the challenge?

And here's the best bit. Just as you can use the 20:30:30:20 guide for GDAs and your food intake, you can do a similar thing for your 30 minutes of activity. You can choose to do 10:10:10 minutes, 5:20:5 minutes or 15:15 minutes. That is, you can take your exercise all in one go, or in three segments of different time lengths throughout the day – it's entirely up to you. Two lots of 15 minutes of brisk walking will do you just as much good as one lot of 30 minutes. It's the fact that you're doing it and, most importantly, doing it every day that matters.

Just 30 minutes' brisk activity every day will do a lot to move you towards your goals. It will encourage your body to make new lean, muscle tissue, which means your metabolic rate will speed up and you'll burn more calories even when you're asleep.

THE MOVING ON UP CHALLENGE

So are you ready? Now is the moment to commit to fitting in 30 minutes' brisk walking every day. If you don't fancy walking, try cycling, swimming or dancing the can-can – whatever floats your boat! The point is that you need to introduce more activity on top of your existing day-to-day routine. If you commit to doing something new, with a definite start date and time and another date to evaluate your progress, you're far more likely to do it and stick to it.

That's it! It's as simple as that – put on your trainers and start walking.

Ask yourself

Could you:

▶ Walk to work, or part of the way?
▶ Walk the kids to school?
▶ Cancel the papers and go and collect them yourself?
▶ Get out of the office at lunchtime?
▶ Take a walk when you get in from work?
▶ Get the kids away from the TV or computer and walk with them?
▶ Walk the dog, or someone else's dog?

Every step you take will help you towards becoming more active and take you one step closer to the health and weight management benefits that prompted you to read this book. The best news is, you *will* start to feel those benefits *very quickly*. Your body will soon notice that you're asking it to do more than usual, and that's when the changes will start to happen. Your metabolic rate will improve, and therefore your efficiency at burning calories and your ability to lose weight will also improve. Once you start to make progress, you're much less likely to want to put it at risk by eating extra fatty foods and biscuits.

If you're stuck for time and not sure where you can find another 30 minutes in your day, start by looking at your current routine and see when you could walk instead of driving or taking the bus, or watching TV. There are always choices to be made.

You might find it useful to plan a couple of walking circuits that will take you 10, 15 or 30 minutes to complete, so you don't have to think about where you're going to walk. Make sure you feel safe and, if you're worried about any existing health problems, check with your doctor first.

THE PROS AND CONS OF GETTING A MOVE ON

Whenever you're contemplating starting something new, there are always pros and cons, and sometimes the cons have a niggling habit of stopping you from getting started. If you know what the cons are before you start, make sure you have the answers against them ready in your head, so you can see them off when they try to tell you not to bother.

'I love the idea of being active rather than exercising. By combining activity with my healthy GDA Diet I've lost over a stone and dropped from a size 14 to a 12.'
Penny T, Essex

Of course, the pros should always outweigh the cons. As soon as you're clear about why becoming more active is important to you, you will have a point of focus, the effort you need to get started will reduce, and the activity will appear all the more worthwhile because you'll feel motivated to succeed.

Here are some tactics for seeing off the negative voice that prevents you from starting your new way of life:

Pros	Cons	Bottom line
Feel fitter	It's hard work	Your 'cons' are telling you how unfit you are. It will get easier and easier every day.
Lose weight	It's raining	That's life! Enjoy the fresh air. Buy a raincoat or an umbrella.
Lose inches	I feel silly	What's sillier: worrying about what other people think or doing something really positive to change your life?
Feel more toned	I haven't got time	What else takes you 30 minutes? Ironing three shirts, cleaning the bathroom, watching a soap on TV? Which one is more life changing? Rethink your priorities.
Less breathless	I haven't lost a stone in a week	Fast weight loss is unsafe and you'd almost certainly regain the weight you had lost if you went on a crash diet. It took a long time to put the weight on, and it's going to take a while to lose it permanently.

The key to moving on up and becoming more active is to focus on trying to use up more lifestyle calories – that's calories you can burn just by doing daily activities such as walking to the shops or work, using stairs instead of a lift.

This chart shows just how many calories an hour you can burn off doing everyday activities, depending on your current weight.

Weight	Activity	Calories per hour
65 kg (10 stone)	Cycling 16–19 mph	864
90 kg (14 stone)		1152
65 kg (10 stone)	Running 5 miles per hour	576
90 kg (14 stone)		768
65 kg (10 stone)	Brisk walk/jog at 3.5 miles per hour	288
90 kg (14 stone)		384
65 kg (10 stone)	Dancing (disco, salsa)	396
90 kg (14 stone)		528
65 kg (10 stone)	Digging garden	320
90 kg (14 stone)		445
65 kg (10 stone)	Low-impact aerobics class	320
90 kg (14 stone)		445
65 kg (10 stone)	Step aerobics	540
90 kg (14 stone)		757
65 kg (10 stone)	Washing car	190
90 kg (14 stone)		267
65 kg (10 stone)	Vacuuming	220
90 kg (14 stone)		311
65 kg (10 stone)	Leisurely swim	381
90 kg (14 stone)		534
65 kg (10 stone)	Sweeping leaves	250
90 kg (14 stone)		356
65 kg (10 stone)	Yoga	159
90 kg (14 stone)		222

Regular activity results in your body becoming more efficient at burning calories – 24 hours a day, 7 days a week!

An alternative way to measure how far you are walking, and how well you are doing, is to wear a pedometer or step counter. They are really easy to use and you can get them from sports shops and pharmacies. A kilometre of walking equates to about 2000 steps. Studies have shown that some people find counting their steps much more motivational than watching the clock. As far as I'm concerned you should use whatever method you prefer to keep a track of your walking.

Have a look and see where you come in on my stepometer table. If you think you can do a little more to move on up to the next level, these ideas might be just the ticket to get you started.

Steps per day for different activity levels

Steps per day	Activity level	I say
Under 5000	Sedentary	Only another 1½ kilometres will take you up to the next level
5000–7499	Average	Who wants to be average? Come on, go that extra mile!
7599–9999	Above average	2 kilometres, that's great. Just 20 minutes' walking at lunchtime and you've made it to the 10,000 mark.
Over 10,000	Active	Fantastic, you're doing just fine, but of course there's always room for that little bit more improvement.

Steps per day	Activity level	I say
Over 12,000	Highly active	I take my hat and walking boots off to you – you're a great example to us all. Well done!

'I thought I'd never find time to fit in more walking with my job, but using the pedometer really keeps me focused. I get a real kick out of seeing another 500 steps here and 300 there. It soon mounts up.'
Tony F, London

MAKING A DIFFERENCE

In my clinics, guess when most women tell me they remember first gaining weight? Answer: When they stop walking the kids to school. This comes up so often in consultations. The diet stayed on track, but the 15- or 20-minute walk to school and back every day stopped, which was enough to lead them to pile on the pounds. What actually happened was they removed a significant segment of regular activity from their day-to-day routine, their metabolic rate slowed down and they started to gain weight. Of course, the great message to take from this is that 15 extra minutes' walk a couple of times a day will be enough to see those excess pounds melt away. It really does make a difference.

How do I know whether I'm walking briskly enough?

That's an easy one. A really simple way of judging whether you're walking fast and hard enough is to take the 'talking test'. Start to talk while you're walking (even if only to yourself). If you can talk normally, without getting breathless, then you can probably manage to walk faster or include more of an incline on your walk. If you can still talk but need to catch your breath, you're walking at the right level of difficulty and can keep your pace going. If you can't talk, have turned purple and keeled over, you're probably trying too hard!

Seriously, don't go mad. Start gradually and build up to a level where you start to feel a little warmer and that increases your breathing rate. That level will eventually feel quite normal and will require little or no effort. That's the point at which to up the pace, to see if you can go faster, harder or longer.

What if I can't get about much?

If it's impossible for you get up and about, don't worry. You can still control your weight, but it does mean it will be a little harder for you than for people who can be active. Some people find swimming is a good option because the water, rather than their joints, supports their weight. Chair exercises can also be really helpful. Your GP surgery or local physiotherapy department will be able to give you advice about the specific exercises you can do, and also about special activities available in your area for people with reduced mobility.

FINAL THOUGHT

Now you've got everything you need to get started. You know how the diet works; you know how to make the GDA Diet 7-day plans work for you; and you're ready to start walking towards your goals. Brilliant! So why are you still sitting here? Go and get on with it – and good luck!

1 Decide to become more active, as a bonus on top of your current activity levels.

2 Fit your activity into your day-to-day routine. Journeys to work, the school run or collecting the papers are all good starting points.

3 If it's easier, break your activity into small segments throughout the day.

4 If you have any existing health concerns, check with your doctor before increasing your physical activity level.

5 Bookmark my GDA Diet website, and keep yourself up to date with the latest foods, facts and figures: www.gdadiet.com.

11 STAYING ON TRACK

I've never worked with a client who hasn't had the odd slip here or there and I don't expect I ever will. If it was that easy to bring about change, I doubt any of my clients would bother coming to see me – and you wouldn't need this book!

KNOWING THE DANGER SIGNS

Lapsing, 'having a bad day', 'losing your focus', 'falling off the wagon' or whatever else you want to call it is a perfectly normal part of the change process. It is human nature to forget to have your morning snack occasionally, or to end up choosing something unhelpful at lunchtime. It happens because you got too hungry to make a sensible choice, not because you have no willpower. Likewise, being invited for dinner and eating a meal that doesn't quite fit in with GDA principles is being polite, not weak willed.

A lapse is a slip; a relapse is a return to old ways ...

A lapse becomes a problem when it triggers all kinds of negative thinking: feelings of hopelessness, complacency and guilt. Negative thoughts can turn even a short lapse into a real danger of a complete relapse, and within minutes you can have ended your diet effort and be facing the prospect of starting all over again.

What kinds of comments are the danger signs? Take a look at the following:

- ► 'I've never had any willpower.'
- ► 'I always give in to temptation.'
- ► 'I've blown it.'
- ► 'I'm miserable – let's eat.'
- ► 'I'm even more miserable – let's eat some more.'
- ► 'One biscuit won't hurt.'
- ► 'I'll never lose weight, so what's the point of trying?'

This negative self-talk is the trick that experiences from past diet cycles like to play on us. Your old, out-dated behaviour tries to exert power over the new relationship you have with food. Be patient with yourself. The unhealthy food behaviours that you learnt and honed to perfection in the past have reinforced your negative self-belief. It will take time, practice and small successes to transform these thought processes into a more positive cycle.

If you are to find your way to permanent weight management, then facing negative thoughts head on and beating them is a critical part of transforming the diet cycle.

I want to help you to see a short lapse for what it is:

- ► Understand why it happened
- ► Decide to deal with the situation differently in the future
- ► Move on and let the feelings go – end of story

One of the most damaging thoughts is complacency. It's the voice that says: 'One biscuit won't hurt.' Well, no – in the grand scheme of things one biscuit won't mean you regain all the weight you've lost, and it won't mean that you suddenly increase your risk of heart disease or diabetes. One biscuit is not an international disaster! However, don't kid yourself. When you're trying to build a new relationship with food, one biscuit can lead to two, then to three and then to a whole packet. You can't remove all temptation from every aspect of life, but if you're aware of how you will react if temptation passes your door, you can make sure you're prepared. Let that tempting food stay on the supermarket shelves and never bring it home to tempt you.

Another common mistake that people make is believing that external influences justify losing your focus. The bottom line is that you have chosen to make some very positive steps to change the way you eat and live. These changes will help you stay in control of your weight and keep you on the road to better long-term health. The key message in that statement is *chosen* – this is your choice. It will *always* be your choice. While there will always be external influences that have the potential to throw you off track, *you* make the ultimate choice to lose control or stay in the driving seat.

Common external influences that can throw you off track	*Considerations to overcome those external influences and stay in control*
My son loves double chocolate cookies, so I have to keep them in the cupboard for him.	He's not trying to lose weight (yet), you are! Make sure you have non-food treats especially for you. And make sure you aren't encouraging your son to eat high-fat foods as treats too.
It's my friend's birthday and we're going out for a meal. It's going to be a blow-out!	Do you think your friend only wants you with her so you can both overeat? Surely, she wants you with her because you're good fun and she enjoys your company. Let her know that you're really looking forward to going out, but you don't want to undo all the hard work you've been putting in to get healthy.

(continued)

Common external influences that can throw you off track	Considerations to overcome those external influences and stay in control
I've had such a lousy week at work, I deserve a few drinks tonight	Poor you! Stress at work is difficult and can really get you down. Drinking to unwind on Friday might help you forget about it, but the stress will still be there again on Monday, and high-calorie drinks won't help you lose weight. How about unwinding properly with a massage or, a walk?
It's Christmas, there's always so much food around, but that's what Christmas is about	Just as you've been planning for your GDA diet, plan for the celebrations too. Of course have a few treats, but be realistic about how many people you're catering for and for how long. Work through the celebration meal by meal to minimise the leftovers.

CELEBRATING YOUR SUCCESS

It is really, really important to celebrate your successes, no matter how small they seem to be. You resisted the 2 for 1 offer on ice cream? Fantastic – time to celebrate. You lost 1 kg this week? Fantastic – you're still on track. Give yourself a non-food treat. Each time you reach one of your milestones you deserve a huge pat on the back. Although I've made the GDA Diet as easy as possible, you are the one working really hard to achieve the fantastic results each of your 10 per cent weight-loss milestones brings.

Now is the time to take stock and treat yourself. But instead of treating yourself with a calorie-laden treat, how about one of the following?

► Go and see a film
► Get that top you've had your eye on

- What about a hair cut?
- Try a manicure
- Have a night out dancing on the town
- Plan a weekend away

KEEPING GOING WHEN YOU'VE REACHED YOUR GOALS

I've said all along that the GDA Diet doesn't push for speedy, short-term weight loss, ban key food groups or propose a difficult exercise programme. But what is important is to know when you've reached your recommended target weight. Once you have reached your final goal you will need to stop losing weight and focus instead on maintaining the great shape you're in.

Because the GDA Diet is a way of life and not just a quick 'here today, gone tomorrow' fad, maintaining your weight doesn't mean a return to your old ways – that would just turn your success back into an extended version of the old diet cycle. Definitely not a good move. The likelihood is that by the time you reach the maintenance phase, using GDA labels to CHECK, COMPARE and CHOOSE your food will be such a natural part of your shopping routine that you wouldn't want to go back to the old days of filling your trolley with anything and everything.

In the weight-maintenance phase, you can relax your targets a little when you're eating out. You might choose to have an extra glass of wine (and no, I don't mean binge drinking!) or a portion of dessert, more parmesan on your pasta or a slightly richer sauce with your main course. And why not, you're in great shape and know how to stay that way. However, make sure your treats are occasional rather than at every meal or the weight will start to creep up again.

Choose sensibly most of the time, and have a little of what you fancy some of the time. A small treat every fourth day can work well; alternatively, watch what you eat carefully from Monday to Friday and relax more at the weekend, when you can take more exercise instead. Please, please, don't take this suggestion as a green light to go hell for leather at the weekend. It's a sad but true fact that everything you put in your mouth has an effect on your body. No one can get away with bingeing and then starving themselves to try to make up for their lapse, without the body suffering. That kind of yo-yo behaviour can lead to disordered eating and stands for everything I am against.

Relaxing your diet is fine when you've reached a point where you feel very comfortable with your relationship with food, and when you reach the point where you enjoy the confidence that choosing foods with GDAs gives you. If you don't yet feel safe in letting your guard down, then don't do it yet. Wait a while and reconsider in a few weeks' time. Always trust your self-knowledge and go at your own pace.

KEEPING ACTIVE MEANS KEEPING WEIGHT OFF

Another important aspect of staying motivated and maintaining your success is to keep active. I've stressed all the way through the book that you don't have to go exercise mad to be healthy and lose weight, but it really helps if you can become more active every day. As being active becomes the norm for you and develops into a part of your day-to-day routine, you can be really proud of yourself. You have the ability to become a naturally active person and as you gradually increase your activity levels, so you significantly increase your chances of a longer, healthier life!

Maintaining your activity levels is just as vital as maintaining your weight loss. So when you've reached your activity goals, look at increasing your daily activity level a little further by 10 or 15 minutes a week.

THE WEIGHT MAINTENANCE SAVINGS ACCOUNT

I often advise my patients to view their activity like a savings bank. If you put in regular deposits, you can make an occasional withdrawal and still stay in credit! This applies in exactly the same way with your energy balance. Expend a little extra energy through daily activity, and every now and then you can have a day off without piling on the pounds. Unlike your bank account, there's no overdraft facility when it comes to weight control, so don't be fooled into thinking that an extra circuit around the park once a week gives you enough credit to party all weekend and keep out of the red!

The bottom line is:

▶ Use your common sense.
▶ Start gently with your maintenance plan and find the level that suits your body.
▶ Remember, it takes a lot longer to burn off excess energy through activity than it takes to consume excess energy through food and drink.

'I was so scared when I reached my goal that I'd pile all the weight back on again – but as I moved from the 1700-calorie plan to the 2000-calorie plan I just increased my daily walking by 10 minutes or so. It was such a relief to know that my weight was staying the same. Now if I'm a bit indulgent on a meal out, or at the weekend, I just make a few calories' savings the next day and do some extra walking to make up for it. My GDA Diet really has become a lifestyle.'
Sarah S, Sussex

Now I've given you my take on why we should all eat a balanced diet, I hope you'll agree none of it is rocket science. It's all pretty straightforward, and people like me really do go on and on about it for good reason. Healthy eating really isn't just about cutting down on foods. I hate the idea of food being considered as 'good' or 'bad'. All food is good, and we can eat anything we like as long as it takes its place in creating a balanced diet. So don't wait a minute longer. Start to 'think GDA' and enjoy everything that's great about healthy eating.

GDA DIET SUCCESS SECRETS

1 A lapse is a slip and is perfectly normal – but a relapse means a return to old ways. Don't let your lapses turn into a relapse.

2 Be aware of your negative thought patterns and your difficult days. We all have them, but they don't have to beat us. Remember, you are the boss!

3 Plan for your maintenance phase. You can use GDAs to stay on track and help you to CHECK, COMPARE and CHOOSE your food – for life!

12 THE GDA DIET: YOUR QUESTIONS ANSWERED

Understanding a few facts and the logic behind basic healthy eating guidelines can make it easier to see why we can benefit from making some simple changes to the way we eat. I've talked about the reasons why it's important to moderate the amount of fat, saturates, sugar and salt you eat (see Chapter 4), so this chapter looks at all the 'green light' aspects of a healthy balanced diet: the things we should all try to do more often.

I believe passionately that any weight management plan should include a commitment to eating a healthy balanced diet and taking regular physical activity. It also has to be enjoyable so that you can make it a sustainable, safe way of life – rather than a tortuous ordeal. Time and time again we have seen new diets launched onto the scene that promise miraculous weight loss but seem to overlook the body's basic need to achieve not only healthy weight but also a healthy mind and body.

MAKING HEALTHIER CHOICES

The GDA Diet isn't just about reading food labels to help keep a track of your calories, fat, sugar and salt intake, it is also about making healthier choices whenever possible within the framework of a balanced diet. Here are the things I think are important to be aware of for a healthy balanced diet and lifestyle, and I know they will work for you:

- ▶ Eat three meals per day plus two snacks.
- ▶ Keep an eye on your portion sizes.
- ▶ Have some starchy carbohydrates at each meal. Choose wisely and eat wholegrain cereals more often.
- ▶ Aim for 2–3 protein-rich foods each day. Variety is the key. Enjoy meat and poultry if you eat it, but also have fish and vegetable protein from pulses like lentils, beans and chickpeas.
- ▶ Base your snacks on nutrient-dense foods, not calorie-, fat-, sugar- or salt-dense foods.
- ▶ Eat some calcium-rich food every day: aim for three servings.
- ▶ Drink plenty of fluids. Water, tea, squash (with no added sugar), coffee, low-fat milk, some fruit juice and some carbonated drinks are all fine.
- ▶ Have at least 5 portions of fruit and vegetables every day – the more the merrier and the greater the variety of colours the better.
- ▶ A moderate intake of total fat is OK, but aim to have less saturated fat and more of the healthier mono- and polyunsaturated fats.
- ▶ Limit the amount of salt and salty foods you eat.
- ▶ Try to be more active – aim for 30 minutes each day on top of your usual routine.

By following these guidelines you can be sure that you get all the good nutrition you need to look after your body and of course your waistline.

Most of us know about the basics of healthy eating; however, trying to make sure we're eating enough of the things that are 'good' for us and not too much of the things that are 'not so good' for us all of the time can feel daunting. So sometimes we put our head in the sand, ignore the good advice and carry on regardless. That's exactly the moment when the GDAs come into their own.

They help to keep you on track. GDAs aren't about banning or demonising any foods – they are a tool to help you know what's inside your food, keep an eye on some of the not-so-good things, and make an informed choice about what you eat.

To help you, all of the eating plans featured in the GDA Diet show you how to mix your foods throughout the day to achieve a healthy diet as well as a nutritional balance.

Remember that the plans are not there to tell you what you *must* eat; they are simply tools to demonstrate how to put everything I have talked about in the book into practice. If you want to follow them to the letter to help you get started, that's great. But, if you feel confident to use GDAs and my other guidelines to create your own eating plan from day one, then go for it!

BUT WHAT ABOUT ?

By now you will have a number of questions. This section answers the ones that pop up most commonly among people who are new to the GDA Diet.

Should I just eat as few calories as possible if I want to lose weight?

► Absolutely not. Remember, this is not a crash or fad diet, it's a healthy diet to help you lose weight.

► If you eat foods with fewer calories than your body needs or too many foods with 'empty' calories, such as sugary or fatty foods, your body won't get all the nutritional goodies you need every day like vitamins and minerals that keep you healthy.

► GDAs help you to balance the things you need less of with the things you need more of – and that's how you balance your diet. It really is that simple!

Why 3 meals and 2 snacks?

▶ A regular eating routine will help you to achieve your goal.
▶ You won't go hungry.
▶ Meeting your nutritional needs is much easier that way.

Why all the focus on portions?

▶ Defining the size of a portion helps to ensure you don't eat too much in one go.
▶ If you're consistent about the amount of food you eat at each mealtime you're more likely to avoid hunger pangs.
▶ Careful portions mean that you eat until you are satisfied, not until you're stuffed!

Why include starchy wholegrain carbohydrates at each meal?

▶ These help you to feel fuller for longer – which means you're less likely to get hunger pangs and reach for the biscuit tin.
▶ Wholegrains are a good source of fibre, to keep your bowels healthy and regular; soluble fibre helps to lower cholesterol and promote healthy gut bacteria.
▶ People who eat wholegrain starchy carbohydrates like wholegrain cereals, rye crackers, oats and pearl barley on a regular basis have a reduced risk of heart disease, type 2 diabetes and some cancers.

Why 2–3 portions of protein-rich foods?

▶ Foods like meat, fish, eggs, beans, nuts, pulses and Quorn™ are good sources of protein, which helps build muscle.
▶ Protein also helps to keep you feeling fuller for longer.

► Eat a variety of protein foods like pulses, eggs, fish, meat and poultry. They all contain the nutrients that help to make your diet more balanced.

Why snack on nutrient-dense foods?

► A lot of us rely on vitamin and mineral supplements to top up our daily requirements. Nutrient-dense snacks like fruit, yoghurts, cereal bars or unsalted nuts and seeds can give us just the nutrient boost we need to ditch the supplements and enjoy more great-tasting food.

► Small snacks between meals will help keep your energy levels up, and some studies suggest you will be far less likely to look for high-calorie snacks that can make you prone to gain weight if you have them too often.

► Fruit can satisfy a sweet tooth, without all the calories, sugar and fat you'll find in confectionery, cake or biscuits. It will also help you to achieve your target of 5 portions of fruit and veg a day.

'I've always been a "little and often" eater. I have to have something in the middle of the morning and the afternoon. It was such a relief when Nigel told me that snacking was nothing to worry about. He showed me how to use the GDAs to find the snacks that would keep me going without piling on the pounds.'
Denise H, Buckinghamshire

Why do I need calcium-rich foods every day?

► Calcium and vitamin D are vital in maintaining bone mass and help to prevent the development of osteoporosis.

► Milk and dairy products, or fortified dairy alternatives, oily fish with soft bones, dried fruit and some fortified breakfast cereals, are all important sources of calcium.

- We get much of our vitamin D by exposing our skin to sunlight during the spring and summer months. A few minutes each day is all that is needed.
- Choose three servings daily of calcium-rich foods to meet your body's needs. Examples of 1 serving include:
  250 ml milk
  25 g cheese
  125 g yogurt
  1 small can sardines
  100 g tofu

Why do I need 5 portions of fruit and vegetables?

- Fruit and vegetables are naturally low in fat, or contain healthier fats (avocados and olives, for example, contain monounsaturated fats).
- They contain good amounts of soluble fibre – and can help to keep your bowels healthy.
- Most importantly, they are packed with vitamins, minerals and antioxidants, which help to fight damaging free radicals.
- Fresh, frozen, canned (without added salt or sugar are best) and dried fruits and vegetables all count towards your 5 a day, as does one glass of fruit juice.
- Keeping a stock of frozen vegetables saves on fresh food wastage and means you can have a greater variety at mealtimes.
- The colour of fruit and vegetables is a good indicator of the antioxidants they provide. Green vegetables tend to be good sources of iron and folates; red fruits contain lycopene (a red pigment and an antioxidant); and orange fruit and vegetables provide beta carotene (another antioxidant). Eat a rainbow of different-coloured fruits and veg for optimum good health.

A word about antioxidants and free radicals and why I love fruit and vegetables

Free radicals are the bad guys in our bodies. They are unstable molecules that are produced naturally by the body, but we also pick them up from pollutants within the environment. Free radicals whiz around our bodies causing damage to our cells wherever they go. Damage by free radicals has been linked to heart disease, certain cancers and a whole host of other diseases and ailments.

Antioxidants are the good guys: they are the enzymes that roam around the body counteracting the effect of free radicals. They basically sacrifice themselves to stop the damage to our body's cells. Fruit and vegetables are our best source of antioxidant vitamins and minerals and that's the most important reason to aim for 5 portions a day.

A portion of fruit is:

▶ ½ grapefruit or a slice of larger fruit like melon and pineapple
▶ 1 medium-sized fresh fruit, e.g. apple, banana, pear, orange
▶ 2–3 smaller fruit, e.g. plums, apricots, satsumas, kiwi fruit
▶ 1 handful of grapes, berries and cherries
▶ 3 heaped tbsp of stewed or tinned fruit (in juice not syrup)
▶ 1 small glass of unsweetened fruit juice (150 ml)
▶ 1 tbsp dried fruit, e.g. prunes, apricots, apple rings

A portion of vegetables is:

▶ 3 heaped tbsp cooked vegetables, e.g. carrots, peas or sweetcorn

- 1 side salad (the size of a cereal bowl)
- 1 tomato or 7 cherry tomatoes

Why is fluid so important?

- Water is essential for life. Each of us is made up of around 60 per cent water and we can survive only a few days without it. (We can survive several weeks without food.)
- Drinks like tea, filter and instant coffee, no-added-sugar squash, low-fat milk, some fruit juice and some carbonated drinks all count towards your daily fluid intake.
- The nutrients from our food are transported around the body by water and most of the chemical reactions that go on in the body need water.
- Waste products are removed from the body using water; without it we cannot get rid of waste products properly and they build up in the body.
- Water also helps to keep our body at the right temperature. We constantly lose water by breathing and through sweat; if we don't replace it, we're in danger of overheating.
- A lot of people don't even realise they are dehydrated, because they have become so used to feeling below their best. Dehydration can leave you feeling tired, constipated and nauseous and can result in frequent headaches.
- A good way of knowing whether you're drinking enough is by the colour of your urine. If it's pale and straw coloured you're OK; any darker and you would probably benefit from drinking more.
- Most of us need around 6–8 cups or glasses of fluid each day to keep the balance right. In hotter climates this amount increases. Likewise, if we take part in strenuous exercise we need more water than usual to help us keep

cool. A good guide is to drink one litre of extra water for every hour of strenuous exercise.

► Don't wait until you're thirsty before drinking – you're already dehydrated by then.

Why, oh why do I need to exercise?

You'll only find me talking about 'getting active' rather than exercise, so I hope that puts you at ease. Getting more active is an essential part of your GDA lifestyle and in fact any healthy lifestyle, and here's why:

► Getting active will encourage your body to make new, lean, muscle tissue – which means your metabolic rate will speed up and you'll burn more calories even when you're asleep.
► Exercising your heart muscle and lungs will improve your overall health and wellbeing.
► You'll tone up as well as lose fat.
► The quality of your sleep will improve.
► Activity helps to relieve stress and tension.
► Being active will increase your weight-loss result and make your body shape easier to maintain.

You'll find more about getting active in Chapter 10.

1 Eat three meals per day plus two snacks.

2 Keep an eye on your portion sizes.

3 Have some starchy carbohydrates at each meal – choose wisely and go for wholegrain cereals more often.

4 Aim for 2–3 protein-rich foods each day – variety is the key. Enjoy meat and poultry if you eat it, but also have fish and vegetable protein from pulses like lentils, beans and chickpeas.

5 Base your snacks on nutrient-dense foods, not calorie-, fat-, sugar- or salt-dense foods.

6 Eat some calcium-rich food every day.

7 Drink plenty of fluids. Water, tea, squash (with no added sugar), coffee, low-fat milk, some fruit juice and some carbonated drinks are all fine.

8 Have at least 5 portions of fruit and vegetables every day – the more the merrier and the greater the variety of colours the better.

9 A moderate intake of total fat is OK, but aim to have less saturated fat and more of the healthier mono- and polyunsaturated fats.

10 Limit the amount of salt you eat.

11 Try to be more active – aim for 30 minutes each day on top of your usual routine.

PART IV
GDA DIET
RESOURCES

THE 7-DAY PLAN FOR BUSY PEOPLE: 2000 KCAL PLAN – AT A GLANCE

Calories	DAY 1	DAY 2	DAY 3	DAY 4	DAY 5	DAY 6	DAY 7
Breakfast 400	150g melon 1 toasted English muffin 1 slice wholemeal toast 3 tsp reduced-fat spread 2 tsp jam	1/2 grapefruit 1/2 tsp sugar 50g corn flakes 150ml semi-skimmed milk 1 Slice wholegrain toast 1 tsp reduced-fat spread	80g melon 60g no-added-sugar muesli 2 rounded tbsp low-fat natural yogurt 1 toasted crumpet 1 tsp reduced-fat spread	35g ready to eat prunes 1 sachet instant porridge 150ml semi-skimmed milk 2 slices wholegrain toast 2 tsp jam	60g Puffed wheat cereal 150ml semi-skimmed milk 1 toasted crumpet with 1 reduced-fat spread Large handful grapes	125ml Fruit juice 30g malted square cereal 130ml semi-skimmed milk 1 reduced-fat croissant 1 tsp marmalade	30g prunes in fruit juice 2 (27g) sachets instant porridge 300ml semi-skimmed milk
Snack 200	5 water biscuits 3 tsp low-fat soft cheese handful grapes	1/2 packet mini rice and corn snacks 1 small banana	1 mug instant low-fat hot chocolate 1 Jaffa cake	1 small (33g) flapjack 1 slice fresh pineapple	1 toasted English muffin 1 tsp reduced-fat spread	Small bunch grapes 1 kiwi fruit 4 water biscuits 1 tbsp cottage cheese	1 sliced banana 1 tbsp low-fat natural yogurt 2 tbsp no-added-sugar muesli
Lunch 600	1 *salmon and cucumber sandwich 1 toasted tea cake 1 tsp reduced-fat spread 150ml orange juice	300g *Red Thai chicken soup 2 small wholemeal rolls 2 Scotch pancakes 80g strawberries	1 *egg and cress sandwich 1 banana 1 tbsp low-fat yogurt 1 tbsp no-added-sugar muesli	300g *tomato and basil soup 1 granary bap 4 water biscuits 30g brie small handful grapes	1 *tuna and sweetcorn sandwich 2 tbsp oat granola 1 tbsp low-fat yogurt handful fresh raspberries	1 *chicken caesar wrap 1 banana	*individual char-grilled chicken and pasta salad handful (6–7) cherry tomatoes 5 cm (2in) baguette 1 satsuma

Snack 200	1 banana 1 tbsp low-fat yogurt 1 tbsp no-added-sugar muesli	4 water biscuits 30 g *low-fat pâthcl	Vegetable crudithcls 2 bread sticks 1 tbsp *houmous	4 water biscuits 2 tsp low-fat soft cheese 80 g melon	2 Scotch pancakes 1 tbsp low-fat yogurt a handful of blueberries	2 slices wholemeal toast 2 tsp reduced-fat spread	40 g dried fruit cereal bar 80 g melon
Dinner 600	Vegetable crudithcls 1 tbsp *houmous 1/2 large *ham and pineapple pizza large mixed salad 1 tbsp *fat-free dressing	*potato-topped chicken and broccoli pie carrots and sweetcorn 80 g stewed apple 3 tbsp *low-fat custard	400 g portion spaghetti bolognese a large mixed salad and 1 tbsp *fat-free dressing handful fresh raspberries 2 tbsp oat granola 1 tbsp low-fat yogurt	100 g *broccoli quiche 200 g boiled new potatoes 2 m 80 g servings of vegetables of choice or a large mixed salad 2 *Scotch pancakes	450 g *sausage and mash 2 or 3 80 g servings of vegetables 140 g fruit salad 1 scoop vanilla soft-scoop ice cream	*400 g king prawn and vegetable masala or *chicken curry rice 1 (90 g) wholemeal pitta bread 1 satsuma	3 slices roast beef with gravy 4 tbsp mashed potato 2 m 80 g portions of vegetables 60 g *fruit crumble 2 tbsp *reduced-fat custard

* asterisk   Ready-made meal or ingredients

THE 7-DAY PLAN FOR VEGETARIANS: 2000 KCAL PLAN – AT A GLANCE

Calories	DAY 1	DAY 2	DAY 3	DAY 4	DAY 5	DAY 6	DAY 7
Breakfast 400	1/2 grapefruit 1 tsp sugar 1 low-fat croissant 2 slices wholemeal toast 1 tsp reduced-fat spread 2 tsp jam	50g puffed wheat cereal 150ml semi-skimmed milk 2 tbsp blueberries 1 toasted crumpet 1 tsp reduced-fat spread	3 wheat biscuits 170ml semi-skimmed milk 1 slice wholegrain toast 1 tsp honey handful of sliced strawberries	50g corn flakes 150ml semi-skimmed milk 1 slice wholegrain toast 1 tsp reduced-fat spread 1/2 grapefruit 1 tsp sugar	80g pineapple 60g no-added-sugar muesli 2 tbsp low-fat natural yogurt 1 slice wholemeal toast 1 tsp reduced-fat spread	125ml Fruit juice 11/2 eggs scrambled 2 tbsp semi-skimmed milk 2 slices wholegrain toast 2 grilled tomatoes 2 tbsp sliced mushrooms	Porridge 60g oats 250ml semi-skimmed milk 1 tbsp raisins tossed in 1 tsp ground cinnamon
Snack 200	250ml *mango and strawberry smoothie 1 tbsp dried fruit	1 tbsp *guacamole 3 rye crispbreads 1 apple	**avocado and tomato salad** 2 bread sticks	80g melon 1 toasted English muffin 1 tsp reduced-fat spread	3 rye crispbreads 11/2 tbsp cottage cheese small bunch grapes	2 Dutch crispbakes **lentil and tomato salad**	2 scotch pancakes 1 apple
Lunch 600	300 g *mixed bean and tomato soup 1 large granary roll 1 toasted teacake 1 tsp reduced-fat spread handful grapes	1 *egg and salad sandwich on wholemeal bread 1 bag mini rye crispbread snacks 1 m 40g dried fruit and cereal bar 1 peach or nectarine	1 wholemeal pitta bread *filled* 3 *mini falafel bites* **Greek salad** 1 tsp *fat-free dressing 1 sliced banana 2 tbsp low-fat yogurt 1 tbsp granola	1 large baked potato 2 tsp reduced-fat spread 1 small tin baked beans (reduced sugar and salt variety) 1 tbsp low-fat yogurt 1 tbsp no-added-sugar muesli 1 sliced banana	**Roasted vegetable couscous and houmous wrap** 1 tbsp natural yogurt 2 rolled oats 1 small banana	**Vegetarian niçoise salad** 5cm (2 in) baguette 1 toasted tea cake 2 tsp reduced-fat spread	**Spinach, feta cheese and mushroom omelette** a large mixed salad and 1 tbsp **low-fat vinaigrette** 1 large wholemeal roll 1 banana

Snack 200	Vegetable crudités 1 tbsp *houmous 1/2 toasted pitta bread, cut into strips	1 slice wholemeal toast 1 tsp jam 1 heaped tsp peanut butter	1 slice wholegrain toast 1 tsp jam 1 tsp peanut butter	4 water biscuits 40 g *mushroom pâté 1 apple	12 almonds 1 peach/nectarine	2 tbsp *tzatziki vegetable crudités 4 bread sticks 1 orange	9 almonds 1 orange
Dinner 600	**Nutty chickpea burger** 1 pitta bread a large mixed salad 2 tsp *fat-free dressing 1 banana	350 g *vegetable lasagne a large mixed salad 1 tbsp Caesar dressing 10 g parmesan shavings 5 cm (2 in) baguette 1 satsuma	120 g *broccoli, tomato and cheese quiche 200 g new potatoes 2 m 100 g portions vegetables of choice or a large mixed salad 2 *Scotch pancakes	**Broad bean, beetroot and goat's cheese salad** 80 g (dry weight) brown rice, cooked 1 kiwi fruit	**Spaghetti Bolognese with Quorn™ mince** a large mixed salad 1 tbsp *fat-free dressing 1 large orange	1/2 *margarita pizza (410 g) a large mixed salad 1 tbsp *fat-free dressing 1 satsuma	**Falafel and lemon couscous with a tomato salad** 140 g mixed berries 2 tbsp low-fat yogurt

*asterisk   Ready-made meal or ingredients

THE 7-DAY PLAN ON A BUDGET: 2000 KCAL PLAN – AT A GLANCE

Remember: Italics = value range

Calories	DAY 1	DAY 2	DAY 3	DAY 4	DAY 5	DAY 6	DAY 7
Breakfast 400	100g can grapefruit segments in light syrup 45g cornflakes 150ml semi-skimmed milk 1 slice wholemeal toast 1 tsp reduced fat spread	3 tbsp muesli 140ml semi-skimmed milk 125ml breakfast juice 1 slice wholemeal toast 1 tsp reduced fat spread	30g rice krispies 140ml semi-skimmed milk 1/2 grapefruit 1 tsp sugar 2 slices wholemeal toast 2 tsp reduced fat spread 1 tsp yeast extract	50g can prunes in fruit juice 2 m 27g sachets of instant porridge 300ml semi-skimmed milk	125ml orange juice 1 toasted English muffin 2 tsp reduced fat spread 2 tbsp low-fat plain yoghurt with 80g (defrosted) frozen mixed berries	1 toasted English muffin 2 eggs scrambled 2 tbsp baked beans 125ml orange juice	40g puffed wheat cereal 140ml semi-skimmed milk 1 low-fat croissant 1 tsp jam 80g can grapefruit segments in light syrup
Snack 200	1 apple handful of grapes 3 tbsp natural yogurt	1 [23g] muesli cereal bar 2 small satsumas 1 rich tea biscuit	1 sultana scone 1 tsp reduced-fat spread 2 tsp jam	Vegetable cruditḥcls 1 tbsp *houmous 4 water biscuits	Large handful grapes 4 rye crispbread topped 40g reduced-fat cream or soft cheese	2 tbsp natural yogurt and 3 tbsp oats 1 small banana, sliced	2 slices wholemeal toast 2 tsp reduced fat spread a scraping of yeast extract
Lunch 600	140g can *mixed tuna and sweetcorn 1 tbsp reduced-fat salad cream 2 slices wholemeal bread 1 sultana scone 2 tsp reduced-fat spread 1 tsp jam	1 large baked potato 200g tin baked beans 25g grated cheese 1 *Scotch pancake	200g can *tomato soup 2 bread rolls 1 teacake 1 tsp reduced-fat spread 1 apple	1 *roast beef and horseradish sandwich on wholemeal bread Small salad of rocket leaves 1 sliced tomato 125g pot low-fat fruit yogurt 1 toasted crumpet 1 tsp reduced-fat spread	**Egg and new potato salad** 1 *Scotch pancake	**2 vegetarian burgers** 170g **roasted potato wedges** 1 tsp *tomato salsa or chutney 1 corn on the cob	6 tbsp baked beans, heated 2 slices wholemeal toast 2 tsp reduced-fat spread 1 tbsp natural yogurt 3 tbsp oats 1 small banana,

Snack 200	3 rye crackers 30g *low-fat pâthcl	2tbsp natural yogurt and 2 tbsp oats 1 large banana, sliced	5 bread sticks 1tbsp cottage cheese Vegetable crudities	2 digestive biscuits 1 mug *low-calorie instant hot chocolate	40g bran flakes 140ml semi-skimmed milk 6 sliced strawberries	30g mixed unsalted nuts 1 tbsp raisins	2 Scotch pancakes 60g can mandarin segments in light syrup
Dinner 600	100g *cheese bacon quiche 240g (8) new potatoes a large mixed salad or 2 m 80g portions of vegetables 140g stewed fruit with 2tbsp custard 1 digestive biscuit	1 medium pork chop, grilled 1tsp *apple sauce 3 scoops mashed potato 2 m 80g servings of vegetables gravy 25g milk chocolate	**Chicken and vegetable stir fry** 140g fruit salad	**Pasta bolognese** a large mixed salad 1tbsp *fat-free dressing	1 *individual margarita pizza (or a 190g slice) 80g vegetables as extra toppings (e. g. sliced peppers, onion, mushrooms) a large green salad 1tbsp *fat-free dressing 1 banana	300g *beef lasagne a large mixed salad 1 tbsp *fat free dressing 5 cm (2in) baguette a handful of grapes 1[23g] oat fruit cereal bar	**Beef casserole** 3 scoops mashed potato 2–3 portions steamed vegetables 1 [23g] muesli bar 1 apple

* asterisk   Ready-made meal or ingredients

bold text   Recipe supplied. Please refer to index

italic text   Available in supermarket value ranges

THE 7-DAY PLAN FOR BUSY PEOPLE: 1700 KCAL PLAN – AT A GLANCE

Calories	DAY 1	DAY 2	DAY 3	DAY 4	DAY 5	DAY 6	DAY 7
Breakfast 340	125 ml fruit juice 2 slices wholegrain toast 2 tsp reduced-fat spread 2 tsp jam	40 g corn flakes 130 ml semi-skimmed milk 1 slice wholegrain toast 1 tsp reduced-fat spread 1/2 grapefruit 1/2 tsp sugar	80 g melon 50 g no-added-sugar muesli 2 tbsp low-fat natural yogurt 1 toasted crumpet 1 tsp reduced-fat spread	35 g ready to eat prunes 27 g sachet instant porridge 150 ml semi-skimmed milk 1 slice wholegrain toast 1 tsp jam	40 g puffed wheat cereal 130 ml semi-skimmed milk 1 toasted crumpet 1 tsp jam handful of grapes	6 sliced strawberries 2 wheat biscuits 150 ml semi-skimmed milk 1 slice wholegrain toast 1 tsp honey	125 ml fruit juice 1 egg scrambled with 2 tbsp semi-skimmed milk 2 slices wholegrain toast 2 grilled tomatoes 2 tbsp sliced mushrooms-sautñcled using spray oil
Snack 170	4 small water biscuits 2 tsp low-fat soft cheese Apple	1/2 (15g) packet mini rye crisp bread snacks	2 tsp chocolate and nut spread 1 thin slice wholegrain toast	23 g cereal and muesli cereal bar 80 g melon	1 toasted English muffin 1 tsp reduced-fat spread	Small bunch grapes 4 small water biscuits 1 tbsp cottage cheese	1 small banana sliced 1 tbsp low-fat natural yogurt 1 tbsp no-added-sugar muesli
Lunch 510	1 *salmon and cucumber sandwich 40 g cereal and dried fruit bar	300 g carton *fresh red Thai chicken soup 1 granary roll 60 g strawberries	1 *egg and cress sandwich 1 banana	*individual, char-grilled chicken and pasta salad 1 banana	1 *tuna and sweetcorn sandwich 125 g pot *jelly handful fresh raspberries	1 *chicken caesar wrap 1 satsuma	300 g *fresh lentil and tomato soup 1 small granary roll 1 toasted teacake 1 tsp reduced-fat spread

Snack 170	125g pot probiotic yogurt handful grapes	3 water biscuits 30g *low-fat pâté	Vegetable cruditḥcls 1 tbsp houmous	4 water biscuits 2tsp low-fat soft cheese	2 *Scotch pancakes	250ml *fruit smoothie	2 fingers *Kit Kat 1 apple
Dinner 510	1/2 *margarita pizza (410g) large mixed salad 1 tbsp fat-free dressing 1 satsuma	450g *potato-topped chicken and broccoli pie 2 m 80g portions vegetables handful raspberries *individual meringue nest 1 tbsp low-fat natural yogurt	400g *spaghetti bolognese large mixed salad 1 tbsp *fat-free dressing	100g *broccoli quiche 170g new potatoes 2 m 80g portions vegetables *or* a large mixed salad 120g tin peaches in juice 1 scoop light vanilla ice cream	450g sausages (2) and mash ready meal 2 m 80g portions vegetables 90g stewed apple 1 heaped tbsp low-fat natural yogurt	400g *king prawn and vegetable masala *ready meal or* *chicken curry ready meal [with rice] Milkshake: 180ml semi-skimmed milk 2tsp low-fat yogurt 8–10 strawberries	2 slices roast beef with gravy 2 m 60g scoops mashed potato 2 m 80g portions vegetables 75g *fruit crumble 2tsp low-fat yogurt

* asterisk   Ready-made meal or ingredients
bold text   Recipe supplied. Please refer to index

THE 7-DAY PLAN FOR VEGETARIANS: 1700 KCAL PLAN – AT A GLANCE

Calories	DAY 1	DAY 2	DAY 3	DAY 4	DAY 5	DAY 6	DAY 7
Breakfast 340	1/2 grapefruit 1 tsp sugar 1 low-fat croissant 1 slice wholemeal toast 2 tsp jam	40g puffed wheat cereal 130ml semi-skimmed milk handful blueberries 1 toasted crumpet 1 tsp reduced-fat spread	2 wheat biscuits 130ml semi-skimmed milk 1 slice wholegrain toast 1 tsp reduced-fat spread handful sliced strawberries	40g corn flakes 130ml semi-skimmed milk 1 slice wholegrain toast 1 tsp reduced-fat spread 1/2 grapefruit 1/2 tsp sugar	80g pineapple 50g no-added-sugar muesli 2 tbsp low-fat natural yogurt 1 slice wholemeal toast 1 tsp reduced-fat spread	125ml fruit juice 1 egg scrambled in 2 tbsp semi-skimmed milk 2 slices wholegrain toast 2 tomatoes 2 tbsp sliced mushrooms	Porridge made with 50g oats 240ml semi-skimmed milk 1 tbsp raisins tossed in 1 tsp ground cinnamon
Snack 170	250ml *mango and strawberry smoothie	1 tbsp *guacamole 3 bread sticks 1 apple	**Avocado and tomato salad**	150g melon 1 toasted crumpet 1 tsp reduced-fat spread	4 small water biscuits 1 tbsp cottage cheese 1 small bunch grapes	**Individual lentil and tomato salad**	4 water biscuits 1 tbsp low-fat soft cheese A handful of grapes

Lunch 510	300g *mixed bean and tomato soup 1 small granary roll 1 toasted teacake 1tsp reduced-fat spread	1 *egg and salad sandwich on wholemeal bread 23g muesli 1 toasted cereal bar 1 peach or nectarine	1 (90g) wholemeal pitta bread filled **Greek salad** 1tbsp fat-free dressing 1 sliced banana 2tbsp low-fat yogurt 2tbsp granola	[210g] tin reduced-sugar and salt baked beans, heated 2 slices wholemeal toast 2tsp reduced-fat spread 1tbsp low-fat yogurt 2tbsp no-added-sugar muesli 1 sliced banana	**Roasted vegetables and reduced-fat houmous wrap** 1 tbsp natural yogurt 1 tbsp granola cereal 1 small banana	**Vegetarian niçoise salad** 5cm (2 in) baguette 1 toasted teacake 2tsp reduced-fat spread	**Spinach, feta cheese and mushroom omelette** large dessert bowl of mixed salad 1 tbsp reduced-fat dressing Large wholemeal roll 1 apple
Snack 170	Vegetable crudithcls with 1tbsp *houmous	3 water biscuits 1 tsp jam and 1 tbsp peanut butter	2tsp chocolate and nut spread 1 thin slice wholegrain toast	4 water biscuits 40g mushroom pate	10 almonds and 4 dried apricots	1 tbsp *tzatziki vegetable crudithcls 4 bread sticks	1 slice wholemeal toast 1 tsp jam 1 tsp peanut butter
Dinner 510	1 m **nutty chickpea burger** pitta bread a large dessert bowl of mixed salad 2tsp *fat-free dressing	350g *vegetable lasagne large mixed salad 1 tsp *fat-free dressing 100g fruit salad 1 tbsp low-fat yogurt	100g *broccoli, tomato and cheese quiche 170g new potatoes 2 m 80g portions vegetables or a large mixed salad 2 *Scotch pancakes	**Broad bean, beetroot and goats cheese salad** wholemeal pitta bread 1 kiwi fruit	*spaghetti bolognese with Quorn™ mince large mixed salad 1 tbsp *fat-free dressing 1 large orange	1/2 *margarita pizza (410g) large mixed salad 1 tbsp fat-free dressing 1 satsuma	**Falafel and lemon couscous with a tomato salad** 5cm (2 in) chunk crusty bread 120g fruit salad

*asterisk   Ready-made meal or ingredients
bold text   Recipe supplied. Please refer to index

THE 7-DAY PLAN ON A BUDGET: 1700 KCAL PLAN – AT A GLANCE

Remember: Italics = value range

Calories	DAY 1	DAY 2	DAY 3	DAY 4	DAY 5	DAY 6	DAY 7
Breakfast 340	*100 g canned grapefruit segments in light syrup* 50 g cornflakes 125 ml semi-skimmed milk 1 slice wholemeal toast 1 tsp reduced-fat spread	3 tbsp muesli 140 ml semi-skimmed milk 125 ml breakfast juice 1 slice wholemeal toast 1 tsp reduced-fat spread 1 tsp jam	30 g rice krispies 140 ml semi-skimmed milk 1/2 grapefruit 1 tsp sugar 1 slice wholemeal toast 1 tsp reduced-fat spread scraping of yeast extract	3 wheat biscuits 150 ml semi-skimmed milk 1 sliced apple 1 slice wholemeal toast 1 tsp honey	*125 ml orange juice* 2 slices wholemeal toast 2 tsp reduced-fat spread 2 tsp jam	1 toasted English muffin 1 scrambled egg scrambled with no added butter or milk 2 tbsp reduced sugar and salt baked beans 125 ml orange juice	1 low-fat croissant 1 tsp reduced-fat spread 1 toasted crumpet 1 tsp reduced-fat spread 80 g canned grapefruit segments in light syrup
Snack 170	Digestive biscuit 125 g low-fat fruit yogurt	1 scotch pancake pear	1 sultana scone 1 tsp reduced-fat spread	Vegetable crudités and 1 tbsp *houmous	A large handful grapes 4 water biscuits 30 g reduced-fat cream cheese	2 tbsp natural yogurt 2 tbsp oats 1 small banana, sliced	30 g cornflakes 125 ml semi-skimmed milk Small handful grapes
Lunch 510	1 home made tuna and sweetcorn sandwich on wholemeal bread 1 *Scotch pancake handful of grapes	1 medium baked potato 1 small tin (200g) * baked beans 25 g grated cheddar cheese	1/2 200 g can *tomato soup large wholemeal roll 1 toasted teacake 1 tsp reduced-fat spread 1 apple	Home made sandwich on wholemeal bread 1 slice ham 20 g cheese, 1 sliced tomato, handful of lettuce, 1 tsp low-calorie mayonnaise 100 g canned peaches in light syrup 1 tbsp low-fat yogurt	100 g canned mackerel 100 g cooked pasta shells large mixed salad 1 tbsp *fat-free dressing 25 g pot low-fat yogurt	1 *vegetarian burger, grilled 1 wholemeal bap 1 tbsp *tomato salsa or chutney 2 thin slices (30g) cheese large mixed salad 1 tbsp fat-free dressing 23 g oat fruit cereal bar	200 g *tomato soup large wholemeal roll 1 small banana, sliced 2 tbsp plain low-fat yogurt

Snack 170	4 water biscuits *30g *low-fat pâthc)*	*2 tbsp natural yogurt 2 tbsp oats 1 small banana, sliced*	3 water biscuits *1 tbsp plain cottage cheese Small handful grapes*	*2 Jaffa cakes 1 mug instant low-calorie hot chocolate*	*2 toasted crumpets 2 tsp jam*	30g mixed unsalted nuts	*2 Scotch pancakes*
Dinner 510	*300g *meat or vegetable lasagne large mixed salad 1 tbsp *fat-free dressing handful of grapes*	*1 medium pork chop 2 scoops mashed potato 2 m 80g servings vegetables with gravy 1 *Scotch pancake*	1/4 (75g) *cheese bacon quiche 6 new potatoes large mixed salad or 2 m 80g portions vegetables 140g stewed fruit 2 tbsp *low-fat custard*	**Pasta bolognese** with large mixed salad 1 tbsp *fat-free dressing	*1 individual *margarita pizza (or 190g slice from large margarita pizza) 80g vegetables as extra topping (e.g. sliced peppers, onion, mushrooms) large green salad 1 tbsp *fat-free dressing*	**Chicken and vegetable stir fry**	*350g *cottage pie 2-3 × 80g portions steamed vegetables 1 apple*

*asterisk Ready-made meal or ingredients
bold text Recipe supplied. Please refer to index
italic text Available in supermarket value ranges

THE STORY OF GDAS

Guideline Daily Amounts or GDAs were first established for adults in 1998, originally for use on the back of food packaging. They came about through collaboration between the UK government, consumer organisations, nutrition experts and the food industry, which was overseen by the Institute of Grocery Distribution (IGD). They were based on the Committee on Medical Aspects of Food Policy's report on Dietary Reference Values (London: HMSO, 1991). This government report still stands today as the basis for dietary recommendations in the UK and is underpinned by objective, science-based evidence that has not been superseded.

In 2005 a cross-industry technical group supported by nutritional and academic experts further developed the GDA concept to include additional GDA values for children across different age ranges, and revised the salt GDAs based on targets set by the Scientific Advisory Committee on Nutrition (SACN). A full set of GDA values endorsed by scientific experts was therefore agreed across the food chain.

To begin with, GDA information was included on the back of food packaging, as it still is on many products. Research by the IGD showed that by 2005 two-thirds of a group of 1028 people had seen the term GDA and of those, a further two-thirds understood its meaning. In 2005 the supermarket chain Tesco looked at the idea of using percentage GDA information on the front of its own-brand packaging to show per-portion nutrition and calorie information in the context of the whole diet. When Tesco researched how the GDA information influenced the foods its customers bought, it found that healthy option product sales figures increased, while less healthy option sales figures decreased.

In 2006 another consumer study, the Omnibus Study, found that 96% of respondents were in favour of food manufacturers using a consistent approach to food labelling and 87% of respondents found the GDA labels 'clear and simple'.

The move by Tesco and the positive consumer research led to the launch of a consistent GDA labelling scheme for use across all food and non-alcoholic drink products, so that consumers could more easily and clearly know what was in what they were eating and drinking.

The GDA label, known as the 'What's inside guide', translates the science underpinning GDAs into consumer-friendly information that can be used to make healthier food choices. By clearly showing the content of a product in per-portion values, rather than per 100 g, the GDA labels relate to the amount of a food people actually consume and how much of the GDAs the food contributes.

'One of the single most useful steps in helping someone address their dietary needs is for them to realise that they have to think about all the food and drink in their diet if they want to change. No man is an island, nor is any one meal a success or failure. You can only make a difference if you map and manage all the food you eat.'
Jane Deville-Almond, National Obesity Forum

THE GDA CRITICAL LIST

Guideline Daily Amounts (GDAs) are supported by some of the biggest and best names on the high street. In the UK to date, 72 companies have adopted GDA labelling: 6 retailers, 3 food services, 2 convenience store chains and 61 manufacturing companies:

▶ Retailers like Tesco, Morrisons, Aldi, Somerfield, Lidl and Netto all use GDAs on their own-brand products.
▶ Manufacturers like Bird's Eye, Danone, Hovis, Kellogg's, Kraft, Mars, Quaker, Ryvita, Tate & Lyle and Unilever, as well as many less familiar names who produce some very familiar brands, also use GDA labelling.
▶ There are even hotels and other people who serve food to us who are using the GDAs.

This means that many of your favourite foods will now have the GDAs clearly displayed on their packaging, helping you to keep an eye on what's inside your food and what you're eating throughout the day.

Check out the websites listed below.

Convenience stores
Nisa-Today, www.nisa-todays.com
Spar, www.spar.co.uk

Food services
Brakes Food Service, www.brake.co.uk

Hotels
Novotel Hotels, www.novotel.com

Manufacturers

AG Barr, www.agbarr.co.uk

Albert Bartlett, www.albert-bartlett.co.uk

Apetito, www.apetito.co.uk

Associated British Foods, www.abf.co.uk

Berry World, www.berryworld.co.uk

Bird's Eye, www.birdseye.co.uk

Bokomo Foods, www.bokomo.co.uk

Britvic, www.britvic.co.uk

Burtons Foods, www.burtonsfoods.co.uk

Cadbury Schweppes, www.cadburyschweppes.com

Calypso, www.calypso.co.uk

Carrs Foods International, www.carrsfoods.co.uk

Coca-Cola, www.coca-cola.co.uk

Danone, www.danone.co.uk

Discovery Foods, www.discoveryfoods.co.uk

Dr Oetker, www.oetker.com

Dorset Cereals, www.dorsetcereals.co.uk

Evron Foods, www.evronfoods.co.uk

Findus, www.findus.com

Fresh Retail, www.jamieoliver.com

Gerber, www.gerberjuice.com

GlaxoSmithKline, www.gsk.com

Golden Wonder, www.goldenwonder.com

Hormel Foods, www.hormelfoods.com

Intersnack UK, www.intersnack.co.uk

Kellogg's, www.kelloggs.co.uk

Kinnerton Confectionery, www.kinnerton.com

Kraft Foods UK, www.kraftfoods.co.uk

Liberation Foods, www.chooseliberation.com

Mars UK, www.marsconsumercare.co.uk

McNeil Nutritionals, www.splenda.com, www.benecol.co.uk

Nestlhc), www.nestle.co.uk

Nichols, www.nicholsplc.co.uk

Northern Foods, www.northern-foods.co.uk

O P Chocolate, www.opchocolate.com
Pataks, www.pataks.co.uk
PepsiCo, www.pepsi.co.uk
Premier, www.premierfoods.co.uk
Pro Pack Foods, www.pro-pakfoods.co.uk
Raynor Foods, www.sandwiches.uk.net
Ricola, www.spar.co.uk
So-Good, www.sogood.co.uk
Shloer, www.shloer.com
Sugar Puffs, www.honeymonster.co.uk
Tate & Lyle, www.tateandlyle.com
The Food Doctor, www.thefooddoctor.com
The Real Potato Co, www.realpotato.co.uk
The Speldhurst Sausage, www.speldhurstqualityfoods.co.uk
Trimlyne, www.trimlyne.co.uk
Tryton Foods, www.trytonfoods.co.uk
Tunnocks, www.tunnock.co.uk
Unilever UK, www.unilever.co.uk
Villa Soft Drinks, www.villadrinks.co.uk
Warburtons, www.warburtons.co.uk
Westler Foods, www.westlerfoods.com
Woodwin Catering, www.woodwincatering.co.uk

Retailers

Aldi, www.aldifoods.com
Lidl, www.lidl.co.uk
Morrisons, www.morrisons.co.uk
Netto, www.netto.co.uk
Somerfield, www.somerfield.co.uk
Tesco, www.tesco.com

GDA labels have been introduced in most European
countries too, including Belgium, France, Germany, Greece,
Ireland, Italy, the Netherlands, Portugal, Spain and in some
cases even further afield.

ABOUT THE GDA DIET WEBSITE: WWW.GDADIET.COM

The GDA Diet website has been specifically created to be a one-stop shop, keeping you up to date with everything that's happening in the GDA world. It contains:

▶ **The critical list:** The most up-to-date listing of the manufacturers, retailers, restaurants and other food servers who are using the GDA labels to tell you what's inside their food.

▶ **The GDA campaign:** As GDAs become more widely used across Europe, we keep an eye on legislation and the campaign to have one form of food labelling across the EU.

▶ **The GDA diet forums and chat rooms:** Log in to the forums and chat rooms to speak to other GDA Dieters, share your success and tips and share your troubles with like-minded people. Of course, you can also just pop in for a gossip too!

▶ **The GDA expert panel:** Our team of experts bring a wealth of experience and advice and are there to support you. There are dietitians and nutritionists, celebrity chefs, fitness experts and more. If you have a question or need some advice, the GDA diet expert panel is all you need to get the answers you want.

▶ **The GDA cookery academy:** Video recipe demos, free downloadable GDA recipes, live webchats and more, bringing a world of healthy GDA food to life just for you.

Joining the thousands of other GDA Dieters at www. gdadiet.com is completely *free*. It takes just a few minutes to sign up and become a part of the biggest, most supportive healthy living community in Europe.

'I joined www.gdadiet.com as soon as I started my GDA diet. It was like having my own personal dietitian, home economist, chef and personal trainer – all at the click of a mouse! I've made some great friends in the chat rooms and have even got a couple of my own recipes featured on the site. It's great to know that if I'm stuck, have a question or even just want an idea about what to cook for tea, I'll find all the answers online.'
Rachel H, Worcs

INDEX OF SUBJECTS

Page numbers in *italics* point to the 'at a glance' meal planners

INDEX OF RECIPES

£↓ = recipes from the 'budget' sections of the book
v = recipes suitable for vegetarians